Soft Tissue Revolution
The New Bodywork Paradigm

Soft Tissue Revolution
The New Bodywork Paradigm

Larry Heisler, MA, LMT

BALBOA.
PRESS
A DIVISION OF HAY HOUSE

Scripture taken from the King James Version of the Bible.

Balboa Press books may be ordered through booksellers or by contacting:

Balboa Press
A Division of Hay House
1663 Liberty Drive
Bloomington, IN 47403
www.balboapress.com
1 (877) 407-4847

Because of the dynamic nature of the Internet, any web addresses or links contained in this book may have changed since publication and may no longer be valid. The views expressed in this work are solely those of the author and do not necessarily reflect the views of the publisher, and the publisher hereby disclaims any responsibility for them.

The author of this book does not dispense medical advice or prescribe the use of any technique as a form of treatment for physical, emotional, or medical problems without the advice of a physician, either directly or indirectly. The intent of the author is only to offer information of a general nature to help you in your quest for emotional and spiritual well-being. In the event you use any of the information in this book for yourself, which is your constitutional right, the author and the publisher assume no responsibility for your actions.

Any people depicted in stock imagery provided by Getty Images are models, and such images are being used for illustrative purposes only. Certain stock imagery © Getty Images.

ISBN: 978-1-9822-3036-4 (sc)
ISBN: 978-1-9822-3037-1 (e)

Library of Congress Control Number: 2019908521

Print information available on the last page.

Balboa Press rev. date: 07/18/2019

Dedication
and
Acknowledgements

After a lifetime, my list of family, staff, teachers, mentors, friends and supporters is long as it is extraordinary.

Feel my love and deep appreciation.

I bow to you dear ones

With special acknowledgements for helping directly in the making of this book, David Derr and Jany Sabins, Esq..

To all my beloveds…I thank you from the bottom of my heart, you have given me strength and love supreme.

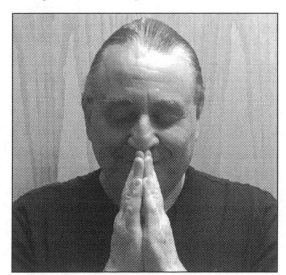

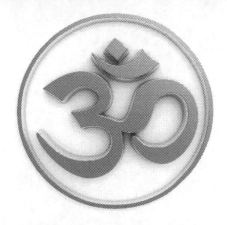

Table of Contents

List of Illustrations

Introduction

When I was in my late teens, I began studying Asian Healing Arts.

It was all under the name Macrobiotics.

The classes I took were not just about organic, locally sourced plant-based eating and natural foods cooking classes.

They also included nutrition theory, oriental visual diagnosis and assessment, macrobiotic medicine and philosophy, acupressure points, traditional barefoot shiatsu, Five Element Theory, Do-In (self-acupressure massage), meridian stretching, chi kung, martial arts, meditation, chanting, sacred sounds, essentially all things yin yang.

When I asked my teachers why we had to learn about meridian energy lines and Japanese bodywork, I was told that shiatsu can dramatically speed up healing by alkalizing the blood stream and boosting the immune system.

I initially had no interest in doing massage.

I was an Assistant Principal in the school system with degrees in counseling and education and later nutrition.

Little did I know how far my alternative education with these amazing Asian and American Masters would take me.

I would be using these teachings the rest of my life.

If you told me when I was in college, initially majoring in engineering, that one day, I would be the founder and director of the longest running school of massage in the State of New Jersey and would eventually teach massage therapy to thousands of students, I would have said you were bonkers.

Yet 45 years later, here we are.

Turned out that the first 8,000 massage treatments I gave were in the style of macrobiotic barefoot shiatsu, I was originally taught.

That turned out to be just a warm-up.

Over sixty thousand massages later, thousands of which were performed on athletes, along with many years of dedicated study in Oriental and macrobiotic medicine, I have the clinical tools and understanding to formulate and share my somewhat unique approach to soft tissue therapy.

There were so many amazing and poignant things I learned from this lifetime course of study that fueled much of my understanding today and specifically about the subject of "How did you get that body?"

I cordially invite you to share in the wisdom I have garnered from my amazing teachers.

The ideas you are about to consider truly is a new massage paradigm.

Nothing short of a Soft Tissue Revolution!

The Fountain of Youth

Why do you think Bob Hope, Rose Kennedy, George Burns and Queen Elizabeth of England called massage therapists their fountain of youth?

All of them said they got or get a deep tissue massage every single day!

For Mr. Hope, he told his last massage therapist, Judy Kemecsei, LMT, that he received a massage every day for 63 years!

She was Bob Hope's massage therapist for 7 years, 7 days a week!

According to these centenarians, deep tissue massage was/is the secret to their longevity.

It does make sense.

> *Deep tissue massage is the secret to their longevity.*

Deep tissue massage prevents the body from freezing up.

It prevents or slows down the arthritis from setting in.

A deep tissue treatment keeps the body soft, warm, pliable, flexible and dare I say it, OXYGENATED.

Oxygenated is another way of saying alkaline and as you might have heard, cancer and many degenerative diseases cannot cultivate in an oxygen enriched environment.

So, you do the math. It's a good jumping off place to begin.

Once an individual's body is soft and pliable, you'll have easier access into the injuries, scar tissue and the energetic system.

Can you say Ponce de Leon?

So Important

One day I bumped into my teacher, the famous macrobiotic diet guru, Michio Kushi. He put his hand on my heart, looked directly into my eyes and simply said,

"Larry, give it all away. The more you give, the richer you'll become."

Then he smiled lovingly and tapped me on the chest and kept walking.

I've tried to do that everyday of my life and I have the feeling that you have too. Perhaps our guru is Hippocrates, known to be The Father of Medicine.

Hippocrates said, massage therapy (The Greeks call anatripsis) should be part of the treatment plan for every complaint and condition.

> *Give it all away.*
> *The more you give, the*
> *richer you'll become.*

Are you a massage, soft tissue therapist or a healer of some sort? If you are, this message is especially for you. What you do is so, so important. The world needs your gifts now, more than ever.

No one does what you do. No one.

A good pair of hands can…

- break up the hardness, the adhesions, the glue that makes us old, rigid and inflexible,
- rid the body of trigger points and scar tissue,
- strip away the fascial armoring,
- relieve pain, lessen suffering,
- open blockages and imbalances in the energetic system.

You oxygenate and alkalize the blood stream that helps in healing and especially prevention. You release endorphins and boost the immune system.

You keep the arthritis from setting in.

You literally reverse the aging process by making us look youthful, even flexible.

BUT MOST IMPORTANTLY…

You devoted your life to compassion and empathy, in touching and improving people's lives and making a difference.

That means we won't have to lie about you at your funeral. You are, a healer in the hands-on tradition. And if you are a massage therapist, you've even taken a vow of poverty.

Shhh…I won't tell anyone.

How Did You Get That Body?

A triathlon like the Iron Man in Hawaii, consists of a 2.4-mile swim, a 112-mile bike ride and a 26.2-mile marathon run, with no rest in between competitions. Back in the late 1980's, I was privileged to work on a fella who was a world-famous tri-athlete. When I asked him how he ate to prepare for competition, he mentioned he as well as many other top tri-athletes were all vegan. I asked him how they all came to the conclusion that an entirely plant-based diet would give them the best opportunity for competitive success, he told me about a German Shepherd study. Apparently, there were two set of dogs. The first set were fed a traditional meat-based diet, the second set a vegetarian cuisine. Of course, when you think of German shepherds with all those canine teeth, you don't think brown rice and vegetables. The first set of dogs were extremely fast off the sprint but after running for a while they ran out of gas and essentially stopped, lied down and panted. The second set of dogs, the veggie dogs, ran slower out of the gate but something remarkable was noticed; they kept running and running. Apparently, their endurance was significantly improved by the vegetarian diet. As athletes started to adopt a vegan diet, they noticed significant improvement in their own competitive times and an important lessening in injuries. As I questioned my tri-athlete more, it became clear that his body was so fine tuned that he would be able to estimate what would happen to his times when he ate an animal-oriented dish. When I asked him, what would happen if he had a piece of salmon, an omelet or a slice of pizza, he explained how much more time it could add to his run, swim or bike ride, making him slower and less competitive. Talk about an amazing fine-tuned athlete, I remember marveling at the notion that he had figured out what effect eating specific foods would have on his body.

Then it hit me! The whole point of this book.

Whatever your personal excess might be (sugar, fat, animal protein, chemical, salt, alcohol, prescriptive, environmental), to a trained eye, it shows up somewhere and somehow on the body.

My tri-athlete said he noticed when he ate something not part of his daily vegan training diet, very often, that specific choice might negatively affect a different part of his body.

When it was a high protein, flesh food, it would affect his back around the kidney region, his hips and the back of his legs. When I asked him how, he said with pain, cramps and increased incidence of pulled muscles.

When he ate sugar, his quads and upper left rhomboid would complain or get knotted or injured.

When he didn't get enough fiber, his lower back and waist would hurt and give him grief.

Suddenly, all my macrobiotic training came into view.

He was talking about the acupuncture meridian energy lines.

Macrobiotic counselors are taught to recognize how dietary lifestyle excesses show up on the energetic map of the human body in every aspect imaginable from your posture and the way you move to the way you express yourself or even how you feel.

In Asian styles of massage like shiatsu, it is said, the pain one feels is a break in the electrical flow.

That pain indicates imbalance in the Energetic (ki) system (acupuncture system).

I teach my students the location of the pain can be the clue to its cause.

Primarily because imbalance in the meridians is caused by lifestyle choices like diet and meridians directly influence the strength and integrity of our muscles.

One of the ways we know this is because of Applied Kinesiology, which is muscle testing.

When a muscle tests week, like the pecs, simply activating acupuncture point Lung 5, directly strengthens the weakened pec.

Ask a quarterback.

Aside from AK, the number one way we know the meridians directly influence the strength and integrity of our muscles is empirically, with hands on knowledge.

You will have to know the Energetic System.

Here's another bombshell.

Excess is reflected in and around the internal organs and all along its energetic pathway.

Whatever muscles lie in the energetic path are directly influenced.

Whether you bounce your legs, sneeze, cough, tear, get pimples, talk too loudly, space out, talk too much, excessively blink, get cramps, sweat profusely, have hot or cold hands, oily skin, eczema, a red, green, grey, pale complexion, it's all about the excess discharging in different ways, from different organs, along specific meridians.

Whichever organ was affected the most by the food choice, its energy line called a meridian would exhibit symptoms.

In Oriental medicine, the meridians are considered extensions of the internal organs.

If you challenge an organ with excess nourishment (more than it could burn), it will also have an effect on its meridian line! So, eating more protein than your body needs will show up in and around the kidneys and bladder and all along their meridian lines. Lats, quadratus lumborum, glutes, hamstrings, calves, Achilles, inside of ankle, all affected.

Excess sugar can affect spleen (pancreas) and stomach meridians.

Fiber or the lack of it, directly affects large intestine.

So, to be clear, I was seeing in real time the negative effects questionable foods have on a finely tuned body.

That got me to thinking.

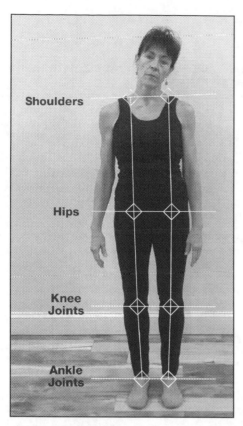

Illustration 1

How Did You Get That Body?

Well, how did you?

Nobody likes to look at themselves in the mirror but when you do look, from a professional perspective, with your trained eye, do you see an aligned body or are you looking at something much different?

Did you ever wonder why a body looks the way it does?

Why your body looks the way it does?

When you watch the news on television, did you ever notice the news anchor with their head tilted to one side?

Why is that? The camera isn't tilted to one side, why is their head tilted? (Illus. #1)

Do you think he or she knows their head is tilting or is it just an unconscious placement?

Here's some more questions.

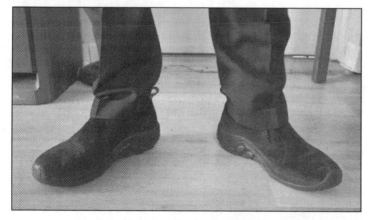

Illustration 2

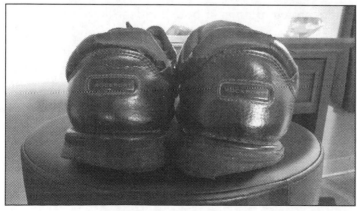

Illustration 3

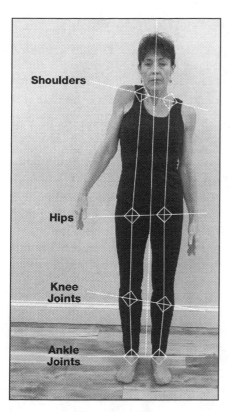

Illustration 4

Do you walk with your feet everted? (Illus. #2)

Do the heels of your shoes wear out to one side. (Illus. #3)

Is your right shoulder higher than the left? (Illus. #4)

Does your waist have a pelvic tilt? That would mean your belt appears on a slant, the back of it higher than the front? (Illus. #5)

How about slumped or rounded shoulders? (Illus. #6)

A lumbar curve showing contracted kidneys? (Illus. #7, next page)

Did you ever sprain your ankle? Was the sprain on the inside of the foot, below the ankle bone or on the outside, just above the ankle bone?

Perhaps a better question…what's the definition of a perfect body?

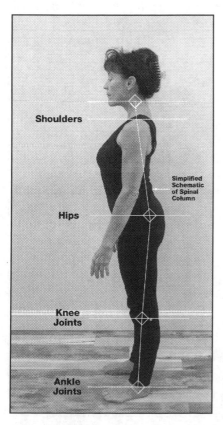

Illustration 5

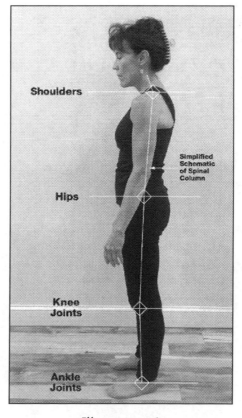

Illustration 6

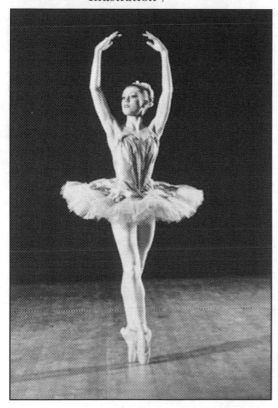

Illustration 7

What does a perfect body look like?

Anatomically speaking, a perfectly aligned body (Illus. #8, #9, #10, #11) is one that shows you standing vertical with your shoulders, hips, knees and ankles all at ninety-degree angles. For most of us this is the way our body presented itself earlier in our lives.

You might have had this type of body when you were much younger but if you're not the prima ballerina, a personal trainer, yoga instructor or an exception to the rule, there are probably going to be what you might deem visible imperfections and clearly defined imbalances when you look in the mirror.

When a person comes to me for a massage therapy session, they sit in the waiting room and fill in the intake form. Afterward, I will invite them to come back into the treatment area. My words will

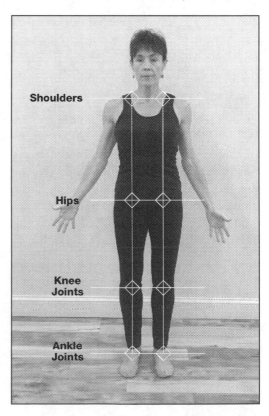

Illustration 8   Illustration 9

usually be, "Let's get started, come on back, please…, after you," pointing for them to walk down the hallway ahead of me. At that point, I observe how they move. I'm taking a general look-see; gait, posture, expression, visible anomalies. That observation, along with their intake history and the verbal communication prior to the session helps me to develop an understanding and then a treatment plan.

But what's the actual cause of all these deviations in posture? I'm pretty sure they were much less when you were younger, no?

First of all, these aberrations happen to all of us, it's not just you.

I guess we can make an argument for many different causes; aging, occupation, genetics, diet, the exercise you do or don't do, psychology (what's eating you), injuries, accidents, illness, surgery, maybe even the mattress you sleep on.

To be politically correct and not insensitive, I will say that using the terminology, "Oriental medicine," is now considered in poor taste.

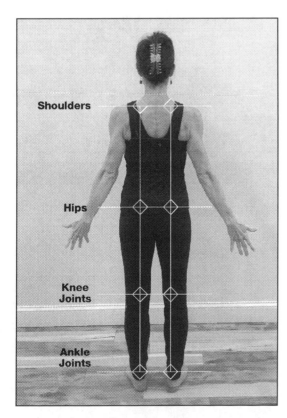

Illustration 10

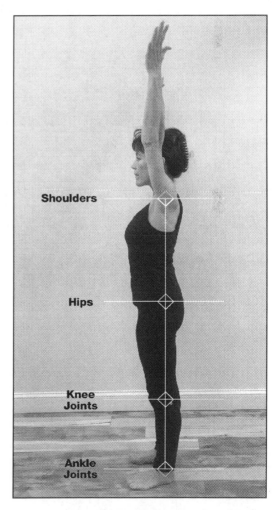

Illustration 11

We are to use the term Asian medicine, but all my teachers who were Asian and especially my main teacher, Michio Kushi called it Oriental medicine. For sanity sake, I will do the same as my teachers.

In Oriental medicine, the hardened, cold, inflexible muscles associated with aging, along with the associative pain and the overall degenerative process is believed to be directly influenced by lifestyle choices and specifically nutritional excesses. My teachers consistently taught, if you consume more than your body can burn or more than your internal organs can handle, these excesses will spill over and affect your overall state of health. That concept will not come as a revelation to most reading this passage, it's almost common sense. After all, we are what we eat and I was always fond of saying "You put junk in, you'll get junk out."

will be a revelation, especially for soft tissue therapists, is the following game-changing concept: the acupuncture meridians, the energy lines that run just under the surface of the skin, are extensions of the internal organs.

If an organ is having a problem, its meridian, and even its acupuncture points, will directly reflect it. That means it can have a direct influence on the condition of your soft tissue. As soft tissue experts, that treat muscular complaints day in and day out, wouldn't it be exceptional to know what influences our patient's day to day soft tissue complaints? That is one of the main premises of this book, exploring the causes of soft tissue problems and not just treating the symptoms.

So, let's break it down…

Acupuncture meridians, the energy lines that run just under the surface of the skin, are extensions of the internal organs.

Symptomatic Versus Integrative

Holistic Approaches

Dad used to tell me if the engine light in the car comes on it could mean my car can have a serious problem. A trip to my auto mechanic or dealership would be in order. Thinking that the problem might be involved is not out of the ordinary. So, if your mechanic looks at your dash and says this will be easy to rectify and then reaches under the dashboard and pulls out the light or better yet snips the electrical wire, you might look at that mechanic in total disbelief. The mechanics approach obviously did not address the cause of the problem. Similarly, if your child gets an ear infection and you take your child to see your pediatrician, you might be given a prescription for an antibiotic. That usually will do the trick. But there are those occasions in a month or two that your child might get that ear infection again. One more time the doc writes a script and now you might be scratching your head. You might even question the veracity of the doctor's action by asking, "Hey doc what's causing my child to repeatedly have this problem? We can't keep giving him antibiotics every time he gets sick." If your pediatrician is a mainstream physician, you might not like the answer to your question. The doc might talk about kids sharing their food and germs on the school bus or an explanation that the child's ear passages are not draining correctly and perhaps a minor surgical procedure to put in ear tubes might be helpful. My kid's pediatrician was more integrative in his approach, practicing what is known as functional medicine. That means attempting to address the cause as opposed to treating the symptoms. When my son would have that specific problem, the doc would say, "No sugar or fruit juice, easy on the mucus forming foods like dairy and flour products and let's give him a dropper full of warm ginger-garlic oil in the ears. Since it took a day or two for the natural approach to work, doc might also recommend some baby Tylenol for the initial pain. While the antibiotics very often work quickly, meaning I would not have to miss too much work, the warm drops and the dietary modifications were a far superior approach, health wise.

When someone comes in for a massage therapy session and they tell you that they have an on-going complaint like an inter-scapular knot (pinched nerve) in their rhomboid, don't we as massage therapists do the same symptomatic approach as the physician? When I teach my Inter-scap Workshop, I give my attendees a protocol that absolutely makes a difference. It combines trigger point work, muscle stripping, myofascial stretching and hot packs. I tell the students to tell their patient, "You might feel much better immediately after I have desensitized the trigger points, stretched you out and used hot packs, but understand by this evening, the pain in that rhomboid might return with a vengeance. I want you to be aware that most of the time it doesn't go away in just one session. Most of the time it will require between four to six sessions laid out in a schedule of three days apart. It depends on how messed up that area is, and like everything else, it doesn't work for everyone. One other very important thing, sometimes the day after a trigger point session there might be some residual discomfort. It is usually nothing more than the charley horse you experience the day after a good exercise class. In my experience the protocol I use can be highly effective."

These successful soft tissue approaches are great, without the side effects of medication, but know this, they do not address the cause of the inter-scap issue. That pinched nerve can and will come back time and time again! So, in effect, the massage therapy we do is just as symptomatic an approach as the doctor writing a script for a problem. As massage therapists, we cannot directly talk about how a high fat diet or a binge drinking session can over-work the liver and gall bladder, weakening the muscles along the right interscapular region. That kind of dietary insult when combined with the wrong exercise, or a bad mattress, or some heavy lifting can create the perfect storm culminating in that pinched nerve.

There will come a time however when we will be practicing functional soft tissue therapy. One that looks at the bigger picture of cause and effect.

HOPEFULLY THAT TIME IS NOW!

Let's start at the bottom of our chart..

The skeletal structure is controlled by the musculature.

Lifestyle

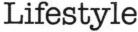

Energetic System: Meridians

Soft Tissue

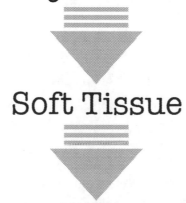

Skeletal Structure

Chart 1, Soft Tissue

In other words, tight, stiff muscles could easily push the skeletal structure out of alignment.

How do we know this? It's in every anatomy and physiology textbook.

Soft tissue (muscles) control the skeletal system.

Therefore, osteopaths (medical doctors that perform manipulation), chiropractors, physical therapists will perform some kind of warming up of the muscles before they manipulate (adjust) your body.

It's also why massage should come before an adjustment, otherwise the tight, in spasm muscles, will push the adjustment right back out of alignment.

You can go back for repeated adjustments and try to train the muscles to hold the adjustment but that might be more about making money than doing what works best.

One of my closest friends and mentors was an Osteopath, Dr. Wally Burnstein.

Osteopaths are taught to warm up a body before they manipulate it.

The techniques Osteopaths learn are some of the most sophisticated deep tissue, trigger point, myofascial work this massage therapist has ever seen.

Dr. Wally showed me a textbook, circa 1940's from the Philadelphia School of Osteopathy. The doctors were wearing suspenders and bow ties and the pictures showed them performing twenty to thirty minutes of techniques to soften and break down the gluey fascia and frozen muscles in spasm.

Impressive work, all done prior to the actual adjustment.

When Dr. Wally would work on someone, it would take about a half hour, all in all.

If you called him for another session because you were still in need, he would say, *"Come back in and we'll hit it again."*

But if that didn't correct the complaint, he would say "I'm sorry this is not helping you," and he would move on to additional courses of action.

Osteopaths nowadays pretty much stopped manipulating because when they do, they can only see two, three patients in an hour.

When they perform general medicine, they can see many more patients and unfortunately medicine is a business.

Dr. Wally would routinely say *"Humans are self-adjusting."*

What he meant by that was, if you adopt and live a healthy lifestyle, your muscles should routinely go back to being soft and pliable and undo the skeletal misalignment (subluxation). When it didn't, he would be there to help it along.

So, to reiterate, soft tissue influences the skeletal structure.

Here's where the chart gets interesting...

You'll notice the diagram shows the Energetic System (meridians) influence the musculature.

We've touched on this earlier.

What does that mean and what exactly is a meridian?

If you've ever seen an acupuncture chart, you've seen a picture with an energy grid that looks like a New York City subway map, all super-imposed along a human body. The lines along that map are called meridians.

The acupuncture system of the human body is sometimes called the Energetic System and represents a schematic of how the human electrical system is laid out. Everyone's system is exactly alike.

A meridian is the electromagnetic energy line running just under the surface of the skin.

While they may seem invisible to the naked eye, sensitive electrical equipment, infra-red and

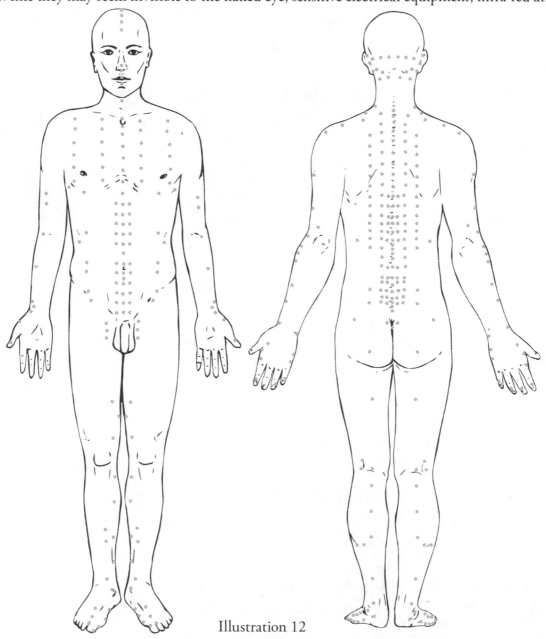

Illustration 12

even radioactive dyes have corroborated their existence. (8)

There is a meridian line for each internal organ and for two specific functions.

There are many names for the energy that flows through a meridian.

In science it is called the electromagnetic current.

In Hebrew, the energy is called Ruach.

In Greece, Pneuma.

The Chinese call it Chi and the Japanese call it, Ki.

The electric current comes down from the Milky Way galaxy and enters our body at the top of the head in a spiral.

The spiral is called a whorl.

My teacher, Michio Kushi says men's whorls run clockwise and women's whorls run counterclockwise

We're going to have to take his word about that.

The magnetic energy comes up from the magnetic core of the Earth and enters our body at the perineum.

Electrical current (yang) runs down along the spine, magnetic current (yin) runs up along the spine.

The two innervate the spinal energy (central nervous system) as well as the internal organs.

Kushi says men carry more electric current (Yang, heaven energy), women carry more magnetic current (Yin, earth energy).

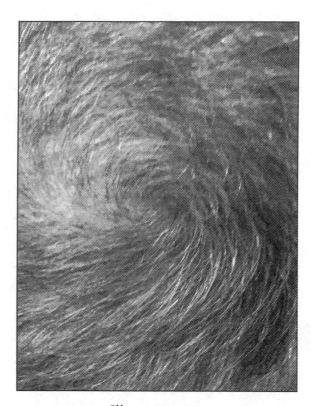

Illustration 13

Now back to the meridians.

There are twelve meridian lines and two channels in the human body (liver/gall bladder, spleen/stomach, lungs/large intestine, kidneys/bladder, heart/small intestine, heart governor/ triple warmer and the Conception vessel up the center front of the body and the Governing Vessel up the center back of the body). Along these channels are acupuncture points my Japanese teachers called tsubos.

There are 360 tsubos on the left side of the body and 360 tsubos on the right side.

Some textbooks say 361, others as many as 365.

These points are entering and exiting points for the Ki.

Essentially access points that allow the practitioner to take out or put in energy.

Treating the tsubos can directly affect internal organs and when applied in combination can be used to treat specific conditions.

Now back to meridians influencing the musculature.

Did you ever see a practitioner do applied kinesiology, known as muscle testing?

It is also called Touch for Health by chiropractors and massage therapists.

They utilize simple tests that can measure the strength and integrity of a muscle.

When the muscle tests weak, there are specific designated acupuncture points that can be activated to strengthen that weak muscle.

Let's say we are testing the pec muscle on a tennis player. You would want the pec muscle on a tennis player to be at its strongest before competition, right? Let's say before the big match, the muscle testing reveals it doesn't test strong. In fact, it tests weak and somewhat compromised.

The point to activate and strengthen the pec would be Lung 5, located above the thumb on the elbow crease.

After Lung 5 is activated (by pressing the point repeatedly), the pec will strengthen and in turn, test strong, leaving our athlete ready for prime time.

That brings us back to our new paradigm that the meridians affect the muscles.

I am the former Director of Nutrition for the medical group my massage school is in. I feel comfortable talking about nutrition, but you should know it's outside the scope of a massage practice. You are not allowed to do this. I'm sharing this insight to make a point.

Some years ago, a gal came in with a stiff, painful neck.

She said the strain was probably caused by the crazy way she sleeps on her stomach and face.

When showing me the painful area, she pointed to the gall bladder diagnostic points on the back of her neck.

I said to her, in Oriental medicine, the back of the neck is associated with the Gall Bladder points.

My teachers taught a tight, stiff neck is sometimes caused by the gall bladder being overworked by excess consumption of specific foods like saturated, hardened fats like cheese and beef, alcohol, strong vinegars, even eggs, and specific exposures to chemicals, over the counter drugs and overeating.

She said, *"I really don't think it has anything to do with that Larry, I think it's just what I said about my sleeping funny."*

"Okay then," I responded, *"Since you sleep so funny, you must get this regularly."*

"When was the last time you had this?"

After some thought, she shrugged her shoulders as if to say, never.

With that I began a line of questioning.

She came in on a Monday and was pain free the day before, so I asked her, *"Tell me what you ate for breakfast yesterday Sunday morning?"*

She said, "We went to the diner and I had a cheese omelet with toast, home fries and coffee."

I responded, *"A diner omelet is usually about four eggs. Did you have any bacon or sausage with that?"*

She nodded yes.

To make a point, I took my pad out and every time she said she ate something that would deleteriously affect her gall bladder, I wrote it down making a loud tap on the pad.

I was attempting to give her a subliminal signal as to the foods she was consuming that might affect her.

I continued, *"Did you have butter on your toast?"* When she said yes, I wrote it down and tapped my pad.

"Did you have cream in your coffee?"

I then carried on to questioning her about lunch.

She shared that they took her son to a neighborhood birthday party.

The kids were in the back-yard pool and the parents hung out inside the house socializing.

I asked, *"Did you consume any adult beverages?"*

She said, *"Yes, I had two glasses of wine."* I tapped my pad.

I then said, *"Usually where there is alcohol, food is served. What did your host serve?"*

She said, *"It was a pizza party for the kids and our host got extra pies for the adults."*

With that I asked, *"How many slices did you have and was it a plain slice or with some topping?"*

Our frozen necked gal smiled and said, I had two slices with pepperoni."

I continued, *"Did you have any birthday cake?"*

She smiled and said, *"They had a Carvel ice cream cake and yes I had a slice."*

All the while I'm tapping away on my pad.

Finally, we got to dinner.

"And what did you do for dinner last night?" I queried.

"We went to an Italian restaurant."

I responded, *"Oh that's my very favorite.*

What did you get?"

She said, *"I ordered the lasagna."*

"Was that a meat or cheese lasagna?"

Now grinning, she said, *"Both actually."*

"How about alcohol?" I added.

"Well we started the meal with a round of Cosmo's and then we split a bottle of red."

I said, *"You guys were having a fun evening. Last question,"* I quipped looking her straight in the eyes, intently.

"What did you have for dessert?"

When she said, *"I had the tiramisu,"* we both laughed out loud.

At that point it seemed clear and obvious, what she had done.

I told her, *"When you are consuming too much saturated fats and/or alcohol in your diet, areas associated with the liver and gall bladder might show signs of excess or discharge. It would stand to reason when I work on the upper right quadrant of the back, where the liver and gall bladder rule, I might find, a hard, cold region in that part of the traps and especially the rhomboids and lats. In the back of the neck there are gall bladder diagnosis points, so dietary excesses very often result in a stiff neck or a headache lodging in the gall bladder points in the temples. Since the gall bladder meridian runs down the outside of the leg, the IT Band and the peroneal muscles might also be affected. From my experience, it's usually not just one thing that creates the situation, it's usually a combination of insults simultaneously that gives us the big physical, muscular griefs. Like a perfect storm, it takes a bunch of things all at once."*

> *Whenever you consume more than your body can burn, that excess will show up somewhere in your body.*

It took two, ninety-minute massage therapy sessions to bring her neck back around; muscle stripping, clearing trigger points, some simple myofascial stretching and deep tissue work to shoulders and back, some moist heat hydroculator packs to neck, shoulders and back.

The simple and effective interaction encouraged her husband, a world-famous athlete to also come in and enjoy some quality bodywork.

Let's review:

Very often it's about excess.

If you are consuming too much saturated fats or alcohol in your diet, areas associated with the liver and gall bladder might show signs of excess or discharge.

It wouldn't just affect the muscles in the back of the neck but anywhere those meridians run.

Excess has a dramatic effect on the body.

It's something that the Western approaches do not consider, and our Western massage modalities don't address.

Excess is a part of every single American's lifestyle, with rare exception.

Whenever you consume more than your body can burn, that excess will show up somewhere in your body.

Something will be hard, something cold, something out of balance.

Which brings us to a short discussion about Oriental diagnosis and its basis in Asian medicine and culture.

This ancient form of assessment is based on observing discernable characteristics you and I readily display.

We can't help it. To a person that understands what you put in your body will create what we see outside of your body.

Particularly when it comes to degenerative problems, imbalances, weaknesses, sickness and visible abnormalities.

Your particular set of excesses, whether they be sugar, protein, fat, salt, alcohol, chemicals, overeating or environmental exposures, all show up.

That is to a person that knows what they are looking at.

My teachers Michio Kushi, Shizuko Yamamoto, Masahiro Oki all had extraordinary abilities.

Folks from all over the world came to them for consultations.

Many found very successful outcomes because the causes of their afflictions were being addressed.

One day in class, Michio was going over the diagnostic pressure points on the inside of the leg.

He walked up to the chair I was seated in and while my leg was crossed, he reached in and pressed my spleen 10 point.

It's located on the inside of the thigh, just above the knee.

With Michio's firm pressure I yelped, *"Ouch,"*

Spleen 10 is a sugar diagnosis point, and sensitivity is an indicator of imbalance and in this case it meant that I had been cheating and eating sweets. Michio laughed out loud and followed up by saying, in his broken English, *"No hope for you!"*

On another day, Michio walked over to me and rubbed my ear.

Between his fingers was my ear grease.

As he rubbed his fingers together, he said, *"You are eating too much fat.*

He Can Smell You from Across the Room and Diagnose What's Wrong with You!

You might have heard of the name Georges Oshawa. My teacher, Michio Kushi's teacher.

These two in particular are the famous Macrobiotic Way of Life counselors and are considered by some, two of the most important integrative medical and nutrition pioneers of the twentieth century.

They received great notoriety for introducing Macrobiotics, a locally sourced, organic, plant-based diet as an alternative treatment option for folks battling serious degenerative conditions like HIV, cancer and heart disease.

> *Simply put...food turns into blood and blood makes our cells and cells make our organs and body. So, we literally are what we eat.*

At the time, the notion of modifying your diet to treat a serious medical condition was considered by conventional medicine, radical and they coined the approach, *"quackery."*

Today, the same plant-based diet is being offered by mainstream hospitals and integrative physicians the world over. I began studying the macrobiotic literature while still in high school and much more seriously while in college. I would regularly travel to Boston to study at the Macrobiotic Study Centers that was later called the famed Kushi Institute.

For a time in the 1970's, New York City had a macrobiotic study center where the biggest names in this macrobiotic integrative medicine taught and practiced. The center was called the New York East West Center for Macrobiotics. This was no ordinary healing center, even by macrobiotic standards. It was a macro center completely women owned and operated by three powerful, visionary women. They came from completely different walks of life, but all studied with the macrobiotic masters and all had a great desire to help, uplift and inspire. You might even know their names from their cookbooks, shiatsu textbooks, education facilities and reputations.

Their names were Serena Silva, Annemarie Colbin and Shizuko Yamamoto.

It was these three gals that taught me a life changing revelation; our blood and our cells are made directly by the food we consume.

Simply put… food turns into blood and blood makes our cells and our cells make our organs and body.

So, we literally are what we eat. Of course, that got me to thinking, what if we eat more than our body needs?

More than our body can actually use or burn? What happens to all that excess? Where does it go? How does it leave the body? Or does it?

Years earlier, Serena, had introduced me to macrobiotic barefoot shiatsu. I must have been 17, 18 years old. I remember lying on her shiatsu mat and her working along the bladder meridian on the back of my legs. When she got to the center of my calves, I jumped from the sensitivity discovered there. When I asked her what that pain was all about, she said, "that's your kidney/bladder meridian. You're eating way too much meat." At the time I was working after school at the first McDonalds in the Bronx. Immediately after that session, I quit the job and became a vegetarian.

When the N.Y. macro center was created, she brought me around to help out and study.

That's when these three empowered women decided to recruit me to teach meditation and healing energy classes at the facility.

All three of these marvelous ladies showered me with love, teachings, amazing healthy organic food and wisdom.

When someone notable was to teach at the center, they made sure I had an entrance ticket.

When martial arts and oriental diagnosis phenom, the macrobiotic master Masahiro Oki was to teach at the center in New York, I was summoned to take his class.

When I arrived at the center, Shizuko pulled me aside excitedly and said,

"Larry…Master Oki can smell you from across the room and diagnose what's wrong with you!"

What does one say to a comment like that?

Whoa?

To me he sounded like one of those amazing Shaolin Temple Priests, with abilities far beyond mere mortals. Movie stuff.

I then talked with Annemarie Colbin, the author of all those famous natural foods cookbooks like the Book of Whole Meals.

She went into a sober explanation that Oriental diagnosis and assessment were a mainstay in the macrobiotic teachings and that this man was an extraordinarily gifted practitioner.

As it turned out, Master Oki was no ordinary human.

There are so many fascinating stories about this teacher but here's a couple highlights:

Oki was a highly trained military spy for Korea during World War 2, a medical and acupuncture doctor that spoke many languages, a master of 16 martial arts who held 34 dans, a yoga master that lived with, taught Oriental medicine to, and learned from, one of the foremost yoga instructors in all the world, B.K.S. Iyengar. Oh, also… Master Oki was a personal student of Mahatma Ghandi. He traveled and taught the world over before creating a Zen Yoga dojo in Japan that treated folks with life threatening diseases. People would come from all over the world to get healthy at his healing center. Oki's style of yoga was called Oki-Do yoga. He modified the routine yoga postures, added martial arts, diet and meditation to specifically treat an individual's personal condition. There are Oki Centers in many countries and his books are written in many languages.

As we entered the classroom, Master Oki was standing in the front of the room wearing what looked like a dark blue silk kimono. The kind with the wide fluffy sleeves that the hands disappear under. Perfect for a martial artist.

He was impressive, with dark intense eyes and in a very broken English welcomed us with a namaste, bowing deeply as he put his hands in a prayer position. In Hinduism, Namaste means, *"I bow to the divine in you"*.

After we got settled in, Master Oki turned to a gal sitting next to me and asked her to come up and lie prone on the massage table in the front of the room. Then the Master put his hands about an inch above her clothed body and slowly moved his hands over her, scanning the length of her posterior.

> *Every area that feels cold all the time is an area that's dying.*

He then exclaimed, *"Every area that feels cold all the time is an area that is dying."*

That one strongly worded statement was a game-changer.

It never dawned on me that our bodies were giving up their secrets.

In this instance, the gal on the table had a cold tush, as in reproductive system.

Master Oki then asked the remaining students in the room to come up and surround the table.

One by one he had us run our hand over his models' body, just like he did. Not touching her body, just allowing our hand to hover above the body to see if we discerned the changes in skin temp as we scanned the body from head to toe and back again. If we didn't feel the cold spots, he would have us put our hand on the actual cold area to feel it.

Then he said, *"The cold spots along the body surface is an indicator of energetic blockage, blood stagnation and possibly a gage of the internal organ condition just below the surface of the skin. It usually comes along with very tight, armored muscles. It's like a frozen zone."*

Master Oki continued, *"The room is warm, our model is fully dressed, why should any area be cold unless it's telling us something."*

At that instant someone questioned, *"Sensei what causes her butt to be so cold?"*

Master Oki then went into an explanation about Americans, dietary excess and the top causes of death. He went on to verbally illustrate.

Excess fat contributes to heart disease. Excess protein leads to kidney disease. Overconsumption of sugar, diabetes of course. Excess environmental exposure, like radiation, x-rays, hormones, chemicals, pesticides, all leading to cancer. In the cold butt instance; hard, saturated animal fat, as in cheese and ice cream. The fat can take hold in the least active areas, like the glutes.

He said one of every three women in America have a hysterectomy by the age of sixty.

A continually cold tush is the early warning system for reproductive disorders.

"Sensei, what about an area that is warm or even hot to the touch?"

Master smiled and then said the now famous word, *"Inflammation."*

An area that is hot to the touch, *"Has a fever,"* he said.

Again, usually an area in trouble or an indicator of excess as in excess salt or meat, sugar or fat.

Another game changing statement!

At this point, the class broke up into pairs and attempted to discover our personal temperature imbalances.

Master Oki then called the class to order, turned to me and said, *"Take off your shirt."*

Grabbing a magic marker, Master made two circles on my bare flesh.

Jokingly he then said, *"I am going to press on the first circled spot, and you are going to have great painnnnnn!"*

With that warning, he pressed the circle he drew on my abdomen along the medial border of my rib cage, around where my liver and gall bladder reside.

In concert with Sensei's pressure, I screamed and recoiled.

Surprised by the shrill of my voice, everyone laughed including myself.

Then Master Oki instructed, *"Lay down on all four's prone on the carpet. Keep your chest on the floor and pick your butt up in the air. Right arm above your head, left arm down by your side. Now take a deep breath and bring your butt down on the left side to the floor and hold it there for a short while."*

When given permission, Oki had me turn over, lying supine and then pressed the spot that was circled.

This time there was absolutely no pain!

Everyone let out a whoa…especially me but Master was not finished and gave no explanation.

This time to make his point, Sensei asked an adolescent child in attendance with his mother to come up and when instructed pressed on my second circle. This one was around my stomach region.

Once again, when pressed, this time by a twelve-year-old, I turned red and let out a yelp.

Master this time had me go through a variety of what seemed like modified yoga postures.

By the end of the routine the circled trouble spot was again pressed and just like the first time, the pain was completely gone.

At this point I required an explanation, so I said, *"Sensei, what just happened?"*

I'm going to paraphrase his answer now.

Master Oki began by saying, in effect, assessment is the key to good medicine.

23

It can also save your life from a martial arts perspective.

To be effective, both require careful observation.

For thousands of years, the Asian cultures developed an understanding about life by observing and taking carefully detailed notes about how nature worked and how it presented itself. They coined the phrase Tao (pronounced dow), which is defined as *"The Way,"* or the natural order of things.

Western medicine is only a couple hundred years old and look how many volumes and textbooks have been written already.

Imagine observing and taking notes about every aspect of life for over five thousand years!

All things which we feel, see, hear, smell, taste and touch can tell us the story of their past, present and therefore their future.

What you have seen me do here today is called Oriental Diagnosis.

It is based on the notion that what you see on the outside of your body is representative of your internal state of health.

At least to a person who understands and uses this system of assessment and diagnosis.

Your bodies condition and how it expresses itself physically, mentally, even psychologically as a human, is the sum total of your genetics, your nutritional intake and the environment you live in and how you live your life.

At that point I had so many questions.

I asked, *"Sensei, what was the pain I felt, how did you know it would be so sensitive and what did you have me do that worked so well?"*

Master Oki then explained, *"You have internal organs that are sagging and have an abnormal placement in your diaphragm. What we did was correct the placement of your liver."*

"But Sensei," I said, *"How did you know my liver was the problem?"*

What he said next floored me. *"Look at your belly button, it's facing to the left."*

When Master saw my blank face he added, *"That's an indication of weakness on your right side. All we did to correct it was to pull your liver back into its proper diaphragmatic position."*

"Sensei, is that all it took, a look at my belly button?"

"Everything that we treated on you today was clear and obvious.

That's what you are here to learn.

HOW TO SEE."

With that explanation, using his understanding of Oriental Diagnosis, Master Oki began correcting many of the visual, organ and muscular imbalances in the students attending the class with simple adaptive yoga postures.

For many, these postures did not have the dramatic effect like on me.

Most were long term projects that required a variety of lifestyle modifications including the exercises along with diet, supplementation and more.

He explained Oriental Diagnosis gives insight into the health of an individual's overall condition, pointing out their imbalances and giving clues to what might be happening in their internal functions.

Since the meridians are direct extensions of those organs, when an organ is complaining, it's meridian is directly affected.

If you know your meridians and how they run along the body surface, you have an indicator of what organ might be influencing the strength and integrity of soft tissue like fascia and muscle.

For instance, tight, stiff shoulders are usually said to be an area that a person holds their tension.

When asked, *"Why are your shoulders so tight?"* an individual might mention that's where they hold their stress or say they do a lot of keyboarding, weight training or to free their hands to work, hold the phone to their ear, crimped up against their shoulder.

If you asked one of my teachers, they would simply say the large intestine meridian runs through the shoulders and tight shoulders is very often caused by a chronic lack of fiber.

At this point in my studies, I couldn't get enough.

I was in a word, *"Voracious!"*

Kushi was a Master of Oriental Diagnosis. He had three books written and dedicated to the ancient art.

Michio said, *"All things which we feel, see, hear, smell, taste and touch can tell us the story of their past, present and therefore their future. No one can hide and nothing can be concealed."*

For thousands of years the Asian culture would keep notes on the visual and observable changes in peoples face and body. The notes would describe how these people's bodies would look or change with the different illnesses or conditions that would come out and how the

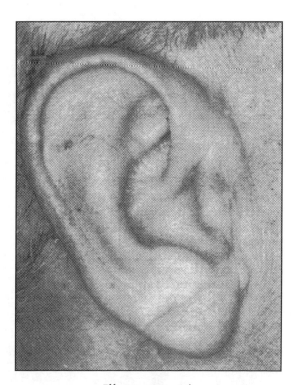

Illustration 14

25

imbalances would manifest on a specific human body and face visually.

Just like the ear crease picture (Illus. 14), signifying an 80% chance of coronary artery disease or a horizontal line on the upper lip, as shown above was traditionally referred to as *"The Line of Woe."* (Illus. 15). This area between the nose and upper lip is considered the area relating to the reproductive system. When this line appears in a woman, Kushi's Oriental Diagnosis states that the uterus has either contracted (too yang) from excess salt, animal food or exercise thus initiating an early menopause, fertility issues, fibroids, hormonal fluctuations or possibly indicating a more serious condition like a cyst, tumor or cancer. With one of three women by the age of sixty having hysterectomies, Kushi would consider this line a foretelling of future reproductive difficulties. In men it's just as serious, an indicator of sexual and reproductive problems like prostate cancer.

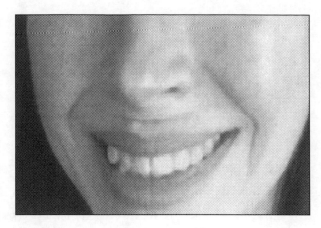

Illustration 15

Again, With the Excess?

America is a country of excesses.

According to Medical News Today, *"Nearly 75 percent of all deaths in the United States are attributed to just ten causes, with the top three accounting for over 50 percent of all deaths."* www.medicalnewstoday.com/articles/282929

It's not a coincidence the top ten causes of death in America are degenerative and have a direct association with lifestyle and dietary excesses.

The top ten are heart disease, cancer, chronic lower respiratory disease, accidents, stroke, Alzheimer's, diabetes, influenza/pneumonia, kidney disease, and suicide.

Sure, genetics plays a factor in everything but like the New York Times bestselling author, Dean Ornish, M.D. says, *"Simple lifestyle changes can reverse most chronic diseases."*

Think about it.

Excessive fat…maybe heart disease, stroke

Excessive sugar…maybe diabetes

Excessive protein…maybe kidney disease

Excessive junk food…maybe accidents, chronic lower respiratory disease

Excessive exposures…maybe cancer

Excessive extremes, excess in general (caloric, dietary, substance abuse i.e. tobacco, non-
    exercise, overweight, junk food, prescription drugs) …maybe suicide, Alzheimer's, immune

Excessive salt…maybe high blood pressure (can lead to heart attack, stroke, dementia)

Excessive calories…

Excessive alcohol…

Excessive prescription drugs…

Excessive acid forming foods…

Excessive chemical, pesticides, hormone exposure…

Excessive ultra violet…

Last one…excessive stress…

Get it?

Oriental medicine and diagnosis are a study of how the excesses manifest themselves and for soft tissue therapists, where?

Let's pick an example.

Do all people with kidney disease display similar visual characteristics?

Oriental medicine says YES.

They've been observing how the human body ages and been keeping notes for thousands of years.

But things have changed as the list of excesses above shows.

Figure you have to die from something right?

Are there symptoms and clues your body gives along the way that will tell you where the problems might be and perhaps clues to what you are going to get when you are older?

Yes! That's the premise of this book.

Learning how to see.

Let's say you die from kidney disease at age 80.

What was happening to you and your kidneys when you were 20? 30? 40?...

> *Simple lifestyle changes can reverse most chronic diseases."*
> *Dean Ornish, M.D.*

Was your body giving you feedback when you were younger?

Kidney disease is the number 9 cause of death in America so it shouldn't be too hard to study closely.

And now that people eat so God awful, with excesses in every corner of our country's affluent existence, it should be even easier.

There are many reasons the kidneys get sick.

The main one, according to Oriental medicine is excess consumption of animal protein but salts, water, over-exertion, lack of sleep, and genetics all contribute.

Keep in mind that animal flesh protein is completely different from plant-based proteins and way, WAY harder on your kidneys.

Flesh food is way up on the food chain.

That's why they are called a concentrate.

As in, concentrated grain.

According to the environmental group Earthsave, it takes 12 pounds of grain to make one pound of beef. (9)

That means the cow must consume the equivalent of about 24 large half pound bowls of brown rice and lentils to make that 16oz. steak.

When we say you are eating high up on the food chain; cows, pigs, sheep, chickens all eat very large amounts of grain to make the flesh we consume.

When you eat the flesh, you are eating concentrated grain and its many days' worth of food in that one steak or burger.

Eating high up on the food chain wears out the body much faster.

When you are eating the plant-based proteins, they are very low on the food chain.

Your body gets all the protein nutrition it needs and without the wear and tear on your kidneys.

THE RULE IS: when you eat more than your body can burn the excess has to be discharged.

Let's give you an example of how the kidney excess might manifest itself and how Oriental diagnosis might help identify it on our body.

When a person eats an excess of protein and salts, specifically a lot of animal proteins and cheap salts like refined table salt, the kidneys must work overtime.

Initially you'll see little signs of the excess discharging or influencing different functions both physically and emotionally.

Symptoms that run along the meridian lines of the kidneys or its partner urinary bladder.

Weakness, heat or cold, sensitivity, cramps, discoloration, pain, ticklishness, specific acu-point pain, knots, injuries, discharge, anomalies, skin eruptions like eczema, etc.

It might not have anything to do with the organs associated with the meridian, but it must be considered.

Things like bouncing your legs while you're sitting. The body's way of releasing/discharging excess kidney energy.

The area under the eyes is associated with kidneys, that's why you get bags under your eyes when the kidneys are tired and overworked.

Generally, it could be from lack of sleep, over working, not giving the kidneys enough rest, drinking liquids in excess or eating too much animal protein.

When the kidneys get tight and contracted from excess animal protein consumption, it will also affect your gait.

When you lie down your feet will splay outward.

Your shoes will begin to wear out at the sides of the heals.

When the kidneys are tight from excess, Oriental diagnosis says you will begin to walk with your feet averted (pointing outward).

Since your quads and hams were created for locomotion, when you walk with your feet averted, your hip flexors are more involved. They are not made for that.

There will be a dramatic increase in chronic hip and back problems, the number one medical complaint worldwide.

In time, as you get older, you'll get knee complaints regularly.

Oriental diagnosis says excess can result in a lumbar lordosis because the kidneys get tight and contract.

You know the frown lines off the sides of the mouth a person gets when they are elderly?

Folks that eat too much flesh proteins and salt get frown lines but over their kidneys.

The next time you go to the beach, take a look at the lines that form over the kidneys. Sometimes it's from weight loss but very often the kidneys are contracted from the excess.

You will have the tendency to sprain your ankles along the kidney points on the inside of the foot.

You'll get an anterior tilt to your waist. Your belt will point lower in the front and higher in the back.

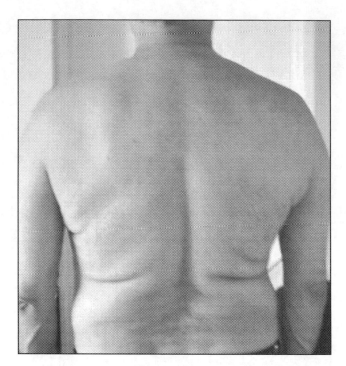

Illustration 16

You'll get more muscular complaints along the kidney and bladder meridians including injuries and cramps when you exercise, especially exercise heavily.

Since kidneys control the adrenal glands, libido, and personal energy levels, initially a high protein diet induces an abundance of energy and an overactive libido.

Females friends consult me all the time about this. They would say *Larry do you think my husband has a girlfriend? He used to follow me around the house like one of those dogs that would hump your leg. Now all he does is watch football and eat. It's like he lost interest.*

Unfortunately, when the kidneys get worn out, fatigue begins to set in, and the libido goes away.

The kidneys control the adrenal glands and high anxiety is synonymous with over-worked kidneys. That along with anxiety attacks, nightmares and eventually depression.

In Oriental medicine depression is associated with struggling kidneys.

Half of America is on prescription drugs for anxiety and depression.

High protein is initially very effective for losing weight and burning calories that's why you'll have so much excess energy.

But then over the long haul, research shows all the terribly negative things that happen like fatigue, clogging up arteries and erectile dysfunction.

You usually won't see the vegetarians slamming around a mosh pit.

And the symptoms go on and on, including emotional and even psychological implications.

In ancient times, traditional martial artists learned Oriental diagnosis. By visual observation they would determine where you would be most vulnerable and attack you there.

Complaints in the organs refer symptoms throughout the soft tissue (fascia, musculature) and a trained eye can see where the imbalances lie.

My teacher Michio Kushi could tell you what stage your cancer was in by looking at your skin and assessing your overall condition visually.

His macrobiotic approach was a major alternative approach for folks battling serious degenerative conditions like cancer and they came from all over the world to engage his expertise. On a couple of occasions, I was privileged to sit in on those consultations and write down the recommendations Michio gave to the patients seeing him.

So let's review our chart again:

Lifestyle

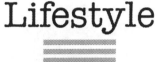

Energetic System: Meridians

Soft Tissue

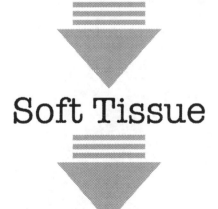

Skeletal Structure

Chart 1: Soft Tissue (again)

Soft tissue can directly influence the skeletal structure.

The Energetic System can have a direct influence upon the musculature.

Our Lifestyle Choices (especially what we consume)

Are You A Practitioner or a Therapist?

If you are still doing the Swedish massage you learned by rote in school, you are a practitioner not a therapist. I know your license says therapist but not just yet. Our profession is in its infancy and there is much to change and improve upon. In the former Soviet Union, a student went to school for five years to become a massage therapist. Six years to become a medical doctor. So, using the word *"therapist"* is a bold statement. My daughter is a licensed professional counselor (LPC). To accept third party insurance reimbursement, which would mean she's the consummate professional in the eyes of the State, the profession and the insurance industry, she needed her master's degree plus an additional 4,500 hours of supervision. She was able to use 700 hours of her internship to fulfill that requirement. The rest was one to one! If you are a therapist, the massage you give me should be completely and entirely different than the massage you give someone else. The word therapy indicates that you have the skills to assess my specific needs and condition and provide my body with a treatment plan commensurate with that assessment. In addition, if I ask you, *"Do you do deep tissue work?"* and you do the same original Swedish massage you learned in school by rote, just deeper, that's not deep tissue work! Deep tissue work is a sophisticated combination of medical massage applications such as muscle stripping, trigger point therapy, cross fiber friction, strain/counterstrain along with myofascial stretching, hydroculator heat packs and perhaps in my case a whole slew of acupressure treatment and pain points. There is no difference between a deep tissue massage and a medical massage in technique. A deep tissue massage is a general overall massage for the entire body. A medical massage addresses specific complaints and issues. For both you need extra education and for the medical, you need more training and practice. A lot more. That brings us to the Ten Thousand Hour Rule.

The Ten Thousand Hour Rule

The Ten Thousand Hour Rule states that to be the consummate professional in any field whatsoever, an individual needs 10,000 hours of experience. Experience can be defined as a combination of school, study, practice and on the job hours. That would be for a plumber, a psychotherapist, an accountant, even a violinist. It's a general rule that takes in all fields. Both vocations and avocations. For massage therapists in the State of New Jersey, full time is defined as twenty, one hour massages a week. With two weeks off for vacation, that's one thousand massages a year. With the five-hundred or thousand-hour curriculum that massage schools offer, to fulfill the definition of the Ten Thousand Hour Rule, it would take roughly about ten years to be considered a highly skilled professional that can deal with any situation that comes your way. Now before you protest, I know massage folks have special gifts. I've seen it my entire career as an educator. Your hands heat up like a bonafide healer and folks constantly tell you about how amazing your work is. I get that. The rule is just a guideline, a generalization. Some of you have gotten to be a consummate professional way ahead of schedule. I'm telling you about the rule because so many in our profession, who are teaching others are woefully under experienced hands-on wise. They might be brilliant instructors and way, way smarter than me on the science side of the equation but nothing takes the place of actual clinical experience in the treatment room. Face to face. Many of my teachers were from Asian cultures, specifically Japanese, Korean and Chinese. For them the word Master means at least 25,000 hours and the word Grandmaster, 35,000 hours and up. So if you do five massages a week for twenty-five years, you would not be considered a Master. Twenty a week for 25 years. Fortunately, there is so much to learn in our field that you can study every day for the rest of your life. I consistently tell folks that I am just starting to get good at this massage thing, even though I'm considered a Grandmaster.

Hardness and Aging

It annoys me when I hear therapists asking their clients what they would like to accomplish in their massage session.

It makes the client think they need to have a reason, a pain, a complaint or some condition to get and enjoy a massage.

Almost as if it is a frivolous luxury.

Maybe the question stems from a poverty consciousness on behalf of the therapist but massage is the fountain of youth!

There are endless benefits to getting a massage.

Not least of which is longevity.

Just by breaking up the hardness, increasing circulation and flushing the body with oxygen, you are genuinely enriching their life.

Part of our soft tissue assessment might be the question, *"Are there any areas you would like me to concentrate on today?"*

If when reading their intake form, they mention a specific complaint, then you might ask, *"Would you like me to concentrate on that area or does that area or any other hurt today?"*

We want people to come for massage very regularly because it is a difference maker.

Word to the wise…

Years ago, Barry came in for his first 90-minute appointment. He was six foot one and roughly three hundred pounds.

The first thing he shared with me was he recently had a consultation with his orthopedic physician and the doctor said he would need two surgical procedures. One for his shoulder (rotator cuff) and the other for his knee. Barry quipped, my doc said he would give me a two for one special price. We both laughed.

I shared with Barry that very often, as we age, we become very armored and tight.

That our fascia develops a lot of adhesions and those adhesions can pull mightily on our joints initiating pain and discomfort.

I also said as I break up those adhesions that pull will lessen and very often the pain will subside and even go away.

About five years have gone by since we had that conversation. Barry comes weekly for his 90 minutes.

So recently, just for fun, I asked him, *"Barry how's that pain you were having in your shoulder and your knee?"*

Barry looked at me a little puzzled, *"What are you talking about?"*

I said, *"Remember when you came in for your first session, you told me your doctor was going to give you a two for one special on shoulder and knee surgery?"*

With that reminder Barry smiled, *"Remember that conversation we had about the fascia?*
"Well…you were right."

Back in the day, I was watching the tennis matches from Flushing Queens. The famous U.S. Open.

Fan favorite, 36-year-old Andre Agassi had won his quarterfinal match. He was so sore afterwards, he had to get multiple cortisone shots to be able to compete in the semi-final match. He was not old by any means but no one his age had won the Open since Bill Tilden did it in 1929. Thirty-six years old for the men's championship was next to impossible to achieve.

As any soft tissue therapist would agree, tennis is a brutal sport on the body. Agassi played valiantly but alas, he lost and after the Open was completed, the great one retired from the sport all together.

I'll never forget how he walked off the court that evening.

I can still see it.

The point of this whole story.

He walked off like he had a frozen back and arthritic hips.

Broken up, like an old man.

As we get older, we get tighter, harder, shorter, stiffer, colder. We get armored!

Did you ever hear the phrase that's used when a horse is at the end of its life?

It is said to be, **"Ready for the glue factory."**

That's the proverbial picture of a horse with the sunken back.

Weird as it may sound, horses like all mammals are good for making glue because they contain a lot of collagen.

Collagen is a key protein found in abundance in mammals and the world is derived from the Greek word for glue, kola.

Collagen is the single most abundant protein found in mammals, being present in everything from horns, hooves, bone, skin, tendons, ligaments, fascia, cartilage and muscle. It's a glue that provides great tensile strength and support.

In humans, collagen makes up approximately 25 to 35% of the proteins within the body.

You know how our attention in the massage therapy profession has turned to *"All things fascia?"*

Well fascia is actually a sheet or a band of connective tissue that's primarily collagen.

So, here's what I'm getting at…

As we get older, we get tighter, harder, shorter, stiffer, colder.

We get armored!

I'm going to make up some words now to make my point.

We become more stickier, more gluier.

Did you ever have a pet that died? Like a pussy cat?

By the end of the day, the rigor mortise sets in and that animals body becomes stiff and rigid.

You can pick it up by the tail and fan yourself. Yes, that rigid.

I know, bad example. But there's an important point.

Just like the horse ready for the glue factory.

For us humans, rigor mortise (postmortem rigidity), sets in way before you die!

I've been saying this one line for over forty years.

So let me say it one more time so you can hear it loud and clear.

Rigor mortise sets in way before you die!

"Rigor mortise sets in way before you die."

You can see the rigidity, the frozen zones, when you watch people walk.

Sometimes even when they are young.

Thus far I have spent 44 years doing massage and have literally worked on thousands of athletes.

For more than a decade, I was doing 40 to 48, sixty- or ninety-minute massages in a week.

I know it sounds crazy, but I had three little children, with a stay at home mother to support and in those days, we didn't get paid well.

I guess in some ways, things haven't changed much. I mean about the *"getting paid well."*

While my observations are anecdotal, they are based on a very large sample size.

So here's a big observation.

The notion of a *"HARD BODY,"* is in my opinion, a misnomer, an inaccurate description.

The only time your muscles should be hard is when you are competing or flexing your muscles.

The muscles of a world class athlete should be soft and pliable.

A tight, hard body is an aging body.

That's why we get shorter as we get older.

Whatever you are doing to get strong, if it makes your muscles short, hard and tight, that's what happens when you get old.

As we age, in my opinion, it's flexibility not strength that's the key.

It's the yogi's that live forever

There are many people, so strong, even on their death bed that can lift me up in the air.

The point here is, *"they're on their death bed."*

Flexibility is more important than strength.

37

My wife Kathy is also a massage therapist and the consummate fitness expert.

She was the former Prima Ballerina of the New Jersey Ballet, choreographed arguably by histories two greatest choreographers,

George Balanchine and Edward Villella.

After she concluded her dance career, she worked with fitness icon, Jack LaLanne and became his number one personal trainer in the tri-state at Bally's.

Kathy even attended the Super Bowl with the great one.

After teaching over 10,000 fitness classes and tens of thousands of personal one on one training sessions, my wife has very specific opinions on conditioning the human body.

Opinions I take very, very seriously and I am sharing with you in this book.

Specifically, when it comes to exercise and training.

Her secret to fitness is to maintain a powerful core and create the elongated, deeply flexible body of a dancer or yogi.

She's on a mission to reverse the current trend that embraces extremely inflammatory types of exercise.

Especially when it comes to educating folks about wearing out their body and the suffering they will experience from inflammation as they age and get old.

Her secret to fitness is to maintain a powerful core and create the elongated, deeply flexible body of a dancer or yogi.

She believes with the correct exercise, never lifting more than two-pound weights, a plant-based alkaline diet, an antioxidant focused vitamin supplement program, regular deep tissue massage and meditation, you'll have the formula for a long, happy and healthy life.

So what does that mean to someone who does bodywork?

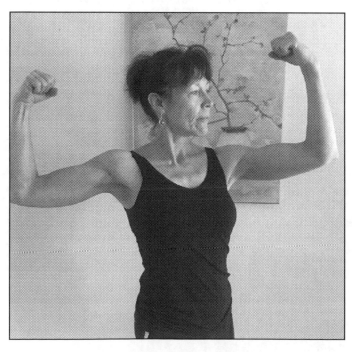

Illustration 17

Our first GOAL as a massage or soft tissue therapist, should be to break up the hardness, TO BREAK UP THE GLUE!

You know how when you take a pregnancy massage class, the instructor will usually cite a handful of acupressure contraindicated points and/or areas not to perform deep massage to?

They might say these acupressure points can induce labor, or should only be performed when you can see the baby's head (crowning)?

Points like Large Intestine 4, Bladder 67, Liver 3, Spleen 6?

My lifetime massage experience says those contraindicated points are much more successful with women eating low on the food chain and much less successful when women eat a predominately animal food diet.

I guess it's a question of armoring. Animal food seems to promote hardness. Plant food flexibility.

Depends on if you eat high up or low on the food chain.

That heavy animal food diet seems to armor muscles, promote tight fascial adhesion and make getting into the energetic flow (acupuncture meridians) much more difficult.

So, for Americans, energetic work like shiatsu might not be so highly effective unless we break up the hardness first.

So, for Americans, energetic work like shiatsu might not be so highly effective unless we break up the hardness first.

Why Massage is the Fountain of Youth

"Bob Hope was my client for 7 years. He got a massage every day for 63 years. Mr. Hope said that a good massage is one of the greatest pleasures in life with many therapeutic benefits."
Judy Kemecsei, LMT Bob Hope's massage therapist for 7 years, 7 days a week!

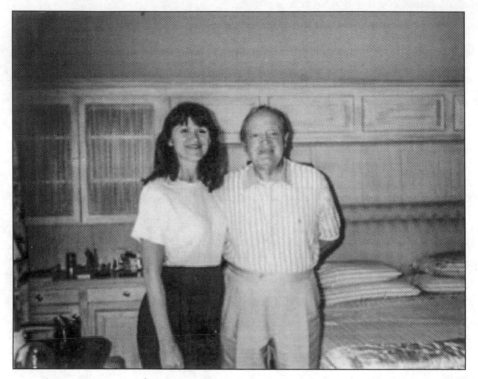

Photo courtesy of Judy Kemensci. www.judykcleansingcoach.com

When asked as they turned 100: *"What is the secret to your longevity?"* Without hesitation they exclaimed, **"Deep tissue massage daily!"**

Think about this.

You are aging. Right now.

What is really happening?

As you age the muscles and fascia shorten, you get tighter, less flexible, less circulation, slower metabolism.

Eventually muscular armoring begins to SET in.

You are slowly on your way to freezing up.

They might call it arthritis, or INFLAMMATION, but it's all about aging.

At what age does this take place? Depends on a lot of factors.

Some you can directly control.

You might have started out at six feet tall.

Only time will tell how tall you'll be by the time you turn 70 or 80.

The glue and muscular rigidity of an aging human body is not too different from an aging horse, as in

"Ready for the glue factory."

For over four decades I've been saying,

"Rigor Mortise sets in way before you die."

During a weekend class at the N.Y. Center for Macrobiotics, my teacher Michio Kushi was in residence.

One day, Michio turned to me during the class and asked me to lay down on the carpet, grab my ankles and bring my heels as far down to my glutes or the floor.

I did as Michio requested and was able to bring my heels effortlessly to my glutes.

Michio looked on approvingly exclaiming in his charming broken English,

"Very good! Many friends are inflexible in their lower back. They consume too much animal food and not enough whole grain fiber. Their choice freezes up the soft tissue over the kidneys, bladder and intestines making them stiff and rigid and incapable of doing what you just did."

To which I responded nonchalantly by saying, *"Well Michio, I'm young..."*

Then with a big grin on his face, this much older gentleman got down on his stomach, grabbed his ankles and brought his heels down alongside his thighs directly to the ground.

A whoa! came up from the audience and then with a big smile,

Michio looked at me and said, *"I guess I am much younger than you."*

Impressed by what I had just seen, I asked, *"Michio, how did you do that?"*

I was thinking he would answer by saying he did yoga or Aikido, something to create flexibility.

Instead Michio looked thoughtfully for a while and answered, *"Ah yes..., Brown rice."*

With that response the audience laughed and Michio continued with his lecture.

I figured he didn't want to answer my question and blew me off by telling a joke.

I didn't realize that he was being deadly serious.

In 1931, the Nobel prize in medicine was awarded to Dr. Otto Warburg. Dr. Warburg discovered that cancer is caused by weakened cell respiration due to lack of oxygen at the cellular level.

He also proved that cancer cannot grow in an alkaline environment (pH 7.36).

Warburg believed that low pH meant lower bodily oxygen levels and high pH meant higher bodily oxygen levels.

Essentially the Nobel recipient spent his life believing that an alkaline body abundant in oxygen was a key to maintaining health.

I incessantly talk about the nutrition heroes of the twentieth century, Michio Kushi and Nathan Pritikin.

When Dr. Nathan Pritikin was in residence at the famed Mayo Clinic (early 1980's), he was dramatically healing what was considered at that time incurable degenerative diseases.

Everything from congestive heart failure and rheumatoid arthritis to insulin dependent diabetes and just about every severe form of heart disease.

In one study, he took a group of men confined to wheel chairs, all in their early sixties.

Blood supply to the legs was so compromised that the average guy could only walk a couple hundred feet before being placed back into their wheel chair.

He put the men on a very low fat, low protein, high complex carbohydrate diet.

They called it the Pritikin diet back then.

Within six months, on this low fat, no junk food, plant-based diet, the results were so dramatic as to be almost unbelievable.

His New York Times best-sellers were titled, *The Pritikin Program for Diet and Exercise and Live Longer Now.*

Predominately a diet rich in whole grains like brown rice, barley, quinoa, along with beans, soups and salads, green leafy vegetables, with small amounts of very lean animal proteins like fish or poultry as side dishes.

It was very strict; no simple carbs like white bread, bagels, muffins, white rice, noodles, no desserts, no sugar, no alcohol or junk food were allowed.

He got the men out of the wheel chairs every hour to walk.

Within six months, on this low fat, no junk food, plant-based diet, the results were so dramatic as to be almost unbelievable.

Every guy in the program was walking six to ten miles a day, most were jogging before the program reached its conclusion.

Their seemingly incurable, irreversible conditions, at least according to the modern medicine of the time, all reversed!

When questioned about the amazing results deemed somewhat miraculous, Dr. Pritikin carefully explained, that with a regular exercise routine, the predominately plant based regimen, would alkalize the bloodstream, raising the oxygen content of the blood within a few weeks.

The improved circulation quickly improved his patient's conditions and permitted their body to start the healing process which was the key to their permanent recovery.

Now here's my point…

Deep tissue massage dramatically increases circulation and oxygen levels just like those miraculous plant-based diets!

Hard, cold, inflexible regions in Oriental medicine is a serious indicator that the rigor mortise is setting in.

A well-trained massage therapist can break up the "GLUE," perhaps slowing, even reversing the aging and degenerative processes of those hard, tight, cold, stagnant, soft tissue areas.

Additionally, once the muscular armoring is broken up, a well-trained massage therapist can gain access into the acupuncture energetic system and literally strengthen the functioning of each internal organ system, boosting immune function, releasing endorphins and generally doing great good.

You might recall that Hippocrates, the Father of Medicine, prescribed massage for every condition and affliction.

So, I am going to go out a limb and submit to you that one day in the future, it will be discovered that massage can significantly help in the prevention of disease and contribute in helping restore a person's health, wellbeing and vitality.

You might recall that Hippocrates, The Father of Medicine, prescribed massage for every condition and affliction.

He knew the concept of increasing oxygen and healing!

That's why folks live so much longer when they get regular massage.

That's why it slows aging and maybe even keeps you from getting some nasty diagnosis.

I believe massage therapy is the Fountain of Youth and we massage therapists are Ponce de Leon!

AND… since massage effects are cumulative, it's also fair to reason, the more you receive, the better you'll feel daily.

You know that euphoric feeling you have when you get up off the table after a great massage. What if you can feel that good every day of your life?

Maybe we should all follow Mr. Hope and GET MORE MASSAGE!

The Difference Between Eating High Up on the Food Chain or Low

Years ago, we got an on-site gig at a Japanese technology company. The middle level management team was comprised of American men. The upper level management team were all Japanese men. The employees had a choice of traditional barefoot shiatsu performed on a mat or a deep tissue massage performed on a table. The American men pretty exclusively chose the table work and as I anticipated the Japanese men chose the mat work. Those of us that got to work on both table and mat had an eye-opening experience. The American men were overweight and displayed an abundance of back, neck and shoulder complaints. The few that tried the mat, complained of neck pain after a couple minutes into the massage. Interestingly, the Japanese men had little problem lying for long periods of time on their stomachs, heads off to the side. Perhaps the Japanese men were used to the shiatsu style of massage, but I believe their bodies were much more fit and flexible than their American counterparts. The Japanese diet at that time was still somewhat traditional. Miso soup, rice, vegetables and a little fish. Meat and dairy products were consumed infrequently. Because the Japanese men ate much lower on the food chain their bodies

Find the hard, cold, rigid areas, and you'll usually find the problems.

were much softer and more pliable. When the president of the company asked to talk with me about the health of his employees, especially the Americans, I felt compelled to fib a bit on behalf of my American compatriots.

That's why I start every session with deep tissue massage, trigger point work, along with myofascial and osteopathic stretching and end with hydroculator steam packs. This singular objective will increase circulation, increase flexibility, alkalize the bloodstream, promote and speed up healing, and seemingly slow down the aging process.

Find the hard, cold, rigid areas, and you'll usually find the problems.

His trainer referred him to me.

When I arrived at the health facility, he was sitting in the waiting area.

The story went like this.

He was just traded to the Denver Bronco's at the expressed consent of people in high places. He needed some serious massage therapy attention as he was nursing a soft tissue injury and his season was about to start.

"So, you're the famous Larry Heisler?"

"Me famous? I don't think so. You're the one that got a personal invitation by the great one. Let's stop b.s.ing and get to work."

There was no intake for this particular athlete.

This was not my main facility and the intake forms were nowhere to be found.

So, I decided to take a verbal history while he was lying on my table.

Before he began to share his story, my hands went exactly to the place that was the source of his grief.

With that simple laying of my warm hand, he sat up and said, *"Whoa, you are good, how did you know that was the spot? Especially before I had the time to tell you?"* I quipped, *"I didn't know it was "THE SPOT,"* I knew it was *"A SPOT."*

"I watched you walk into the treatment room and then while you were lying on the table, I scanned my hands a couple of inches over your body just feeling for the heat variations. My personal experience is that a hard, cold, inflexible area is a troubled area that announces itself loud and clear. That spot was obviously cold and rigid."

There are many different types of bodies; swimmers' bodies, dancer bodies, a yoga body, a weight training body, even a bicycler's body.

> *The only time an athlete's muscles should be hard is when they are being flexed or used.*

Every form of athletic endeavor creates the body that is perfect to compete in that arena.

All have their purpose, their beauty and their practicality.

But the one thing all these bodies have in common is soft tissue.

When you're thinking about a professional athlete, like a tri-athlete or a football player; most people envision an individual that's forever in training and they are.

You think of a body that is perhaps ripped and hard with traps that come up inches off the back in a perfect *"V."*

You think of the proverbial, *"Hard body."*

Ironically, really healthy, seasoned athletes, have muscles that are exactly the opposite of a hard body, their muscles are soft and buttery.

Let me say that again.

Really healthy muscles are soft, fluid and flexible.

In fact, the only time an athlete's muscles should be hard is when they are being flexed or used.

At the moment of flexing they may puff up like a giant blow fish, but otherwise everything stays soft, relaxed and pliable.

So, to reiterate, in my experience, an area of hardness indicates some form of injury or imbalance.

I can be working on someone and everything is beautifully soft and fluid throughout the musculature and then I'll come to that one spot that is hard, perhaps cold and that's *"The Spot,"* the actual reason that person has come to me. Left unaddressed that hardened, rigid area can freeze up and influence the individual's gait and their performance significantly.

Unaddressed in time it feels almost like it's been glued, like one big adhesion.

So, when an average person comes in for a massage, someone who maybe works out but not as a professional, they might present multiple areas under duress; tight shoulders, a frozen neck, an inflexible, cold hip, or even a ropy, hamstring full of scar tissue.

All of these areas are hotbeds of fascial adhesion's, places that freeze up, get old, hard, and stagnant like cement.

If they are not addressed in a timely manner, they will influence the new emerging, imbalanced you.

The senior citizen you.

OH, My Aching Back!

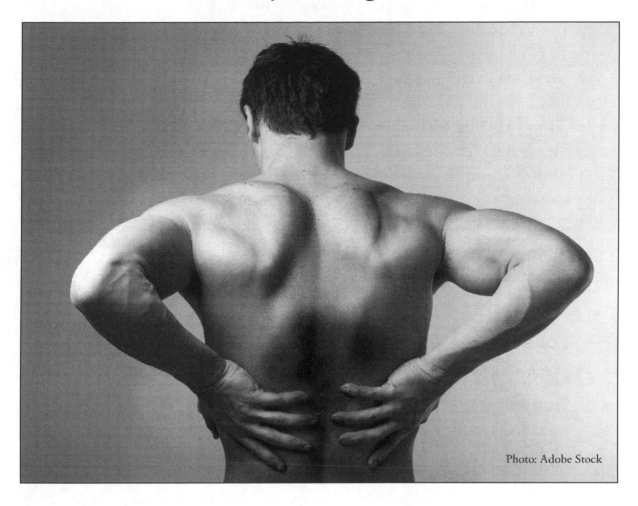

Photo: Adobe Stock

"Back pain is the number one cause of lost work days in the United States."

Dr. Anders Cohen, chief of neurosurgery and spine surgery at the Brooklyn Hospital Center, in New York City.

My grandfather built the Empire State Building, my father built the World Trade Center. My Dad was a bull of a man; Manhattan champ wrestler, a great long-distance swimmer and a champion ballroom dancer, all in a construction workers body. So, it didn't come as any surprise that by the time Dad was in his late thirty's, he was suffering from chronic lower back and knee problems. Throughout my childhood I remember him running from specialist to specialist; orthopedic doctors, osteopaths, chiropractors, physical therapists, physiatrists (M.D. Level PT), all supposedly lower back, pain management specialists. The pain he experienced laid him up for weeks and months at a time and seeing your father disabled was probably the impetus for my massage therapy career. It was time to take dad to see Master Oki, but he had to be prepared because like Oki, Dad had an extremely strong warrior mentality.

I had to explain it to Dad gingerly.

This is how I explained about Master Oki and what would possibly happen.

A revered and brilliant Japanese doctor, a master of 16 martial arts was coming to the macrobiotic center to teach.

His name was Sensei Masahiro Oki and he ran a world-famous clinic in Japan for folks battling serious degenerative diseases.

His skills at oriental diagnosis are so finely honed that he could diagnose your condition by merely looking at you.

Oriental diagnosis traditionally was used by martial artists to determine where their opponents would be vulnerable.

It later turned into a powerful diagnostic tool used by Asian healers and medical practitioners.

Essentially it is the art of observing how an individual look, move and express themselves.

It took your body years to get cold, hard, tight and in pain this bad.

You've run around to every medical professional you could find.

Now it's my turn to chime in with Master Oki.

Dad just nodded yes, and I scheduled the consultation.

> *"You Americans are so foolish, you think you can eat anything."*
> *Sensei Masahiro Oki*

The day arrived, Dad's back was sensitive and hurting.

Sensei took one look at my father and said,

"You American's are so foolish, you think you can eat anything.

Mr. Heisler, the reason you have been suffering so severely is because of your kidneys and intestines.

You hardly eat fiber or vegetables and you are eating extremely too much animal flesh especially beef.

If you don't change your diet, your suffering will get worse.

Your kidneys are very weak and sick."

He strongly advocated dad to consume a completely plant-based diet.

He then hit some acupuncture points on Dads' body and had dad stretch in some very interesting yogic ways and almost like magic, Dad had no pain!

When we got into the elevator my father looked at me and said, *"I think he's full of it, but he did get me out of pain and no one has ever been able to do that, so I'm going to do exactly what he says and see what happens."*

When we arrived home, Dad announced to mom that he was becoming a vegetarian!

Now it was true, my father never ate anything resembling fiber and, in those days, all that mom made was flesh foods and simple carbs.

Eggs for breakfast, some sort of dead thing sandwich on white bread for lunch and more meat, meat, meat for dinner.

A salad would consist of iceberg lettuce and tomato with Heinz distilled vinegar and Mazola corn oil.

Healthy nutrition? No such thought.

After living through the big depression in the 1920's and 30's and then the big war, my folks were just happy to have food on the table.

I think it would be fair to say that Master Oki scared the living daylights out of dad and seemingly overnight he became aware and changed everything.

It's as if the light came on.

The two biggest factors associated with lower back complaints are a chronic lack of fiber and highly inflammatory foods.

He still ate a little fish and some seafood but now it was a macro style diet; grains, beans, soups, salads, fruits, veggies, seeds, nuts, fermented soy products like miso, tofu, etc.

Now here's the really amazing thing;

Dads' consultation with Master Oki was the very last time he had any problems with his back!

What's more, his knee gradually improved and that too never afflicted him again.

On the first anniversary of his meeting with Master Oki and especially pain free living, dad announced to the family that *"Master Oki"* was the most impressive man he had ever met, and he would be eternally grateful to him.

Dad lived another 25 years after that consultation without getting kidney disease and eventually succumbed to asbestos poisoning.

I would say way more than two thirds of the 60,000 massages I've performed have been on individuals with some sought of serious back complaint.

In my professional opinion, after over four decades of performing massage therapy on literally thousands of athletes and tens of thousands of regular folks, it has become glaringly obvious after taking a history, the two single biggest factors associated with lower back complaints are a chronic lack of fiber and, highly inflammatory foods.

Red meat being number one in that category.

Normally I ask each person to account as best they can for the dietary choices leading up to the moment their back became obviously a more serious problem.

I can do this professionally because formerly I was Director of Nutrition Education for the medical group, I still reside in.

Hands down, when I ask what the patient ate leading up to their back pain, I got the same response repeatedly.

Red meat along with a glaringly obvious lack of fiber.

Maybe it's because a pound of beef is the equivalent of sixteen pounds of grain and that's really high up on the food chain or maybe it's the highly inflammatory arachidonic acid in the beef. Allegedly arachidonic acid plays a role in cancer, inflammatory bowel disease and even rheumatoid arthritis.

I really can't say.

Now gathering information like this is called anecdotal or coincidental, but when you've seen and heard the same thing come up *tens of thousands of times*, over forty years, in my opinion, it's not anecdotal any longer, it's science!

The second part to this is equally amazing.

When the person in pain finally changes their diet for good, in other words, when they stop eating red meat completely, they become back pain free for good!

"So let me get this clear, when you got out of bed this morning your back was giving you a lot of pain, is that correct?

And you say you had no pain all weekend but just this morning, something as simple as putting on your pants blew your back out?

Ok, let's think about this for a second, what did you eat yesterday?

What did you eat over the weekend?"

"Nearly one in 10 people across the globe suffers from an aching lower back and in a 3-month period, about one-fourth of U.S. adults experience at least 1 day of back pain.

It is one of our society's most common medical problems."

National Institutes of Health (NIH.gov)

Almost Every Pain We Address Is About Tearing Soft Tissue!

Every time you stretch or bend over to pick up something from the floor or participate in exercise, you are micro-tearing muscle fibers.*(5)

Injuries to soft tissue can happen easily from simple everyday activities, accidents, sports, exercise, and especially repetitive overuse.

The most common soft tissue injuries are to muscles, tendons, and ligaments, which we have an abundance of.

The human body contains 650 skeletal muscles, 900 ligaments and 1,320 tendons.

That's a lot that can go wrong.

The variations in them are in the connections that they make: ligaments connect one bone to another bone, tendons connect muscle to bone, and fasciae surround muscles helping them connect with other muscles.

> *The human body contains 650 skeletal muscles, 900 ligaments and 1320 tendons. That's a whole lot that can go wrong.*

When your client tells you they pulled a muscle or over-stretched, rest assured, it's quite possibly one of these common soft tissue injuries.

Soft-tissue injuries fall into two basic categories: acute injuries and overuse injuries.

Some acute soft tissue injuries are worse than a fracture or break of a bone and overuse injuries can occur over time with repetitive pulling, friction and bending.

Acute can be sudden, as in a mild, moderate or a complete tear and overuse, sometimes referred to as tendinitis, will develop over time resulting in pain and inflammation.

When it comes to sports, 90% of all sports-related injuries are bruises or sprains. (3)

A pulled hamstring for instance, is the most common injury among athletes. (4)

Simply put, a sprain is a tear to a ligament, a strain is a tear to a tendon or muscle.

Do you remember your basic education about how our injuries heal?

An area tears and the body's alarm system goes off kicking on an elaborate repair process.

Unfortunately there is no guarantee that the injury will heal perfectly.

Statistically research has shown the area to be weaker than before.

Scar tissue is the end result of the healing process and in the meantime the area can form adhesions, even high spots in the scar tissue.

It's not like there's someone internally sanding down the rough and uneven edges of the injured area.

That's our job.

Here's the bottom line.

Every time you ask a prospective client where it hurts, consider you are addressing torn and damaged soft tissue.

This quote from Sports Medicine Australia nicely lays out what happens when we tear:

"When ligaments, tendons and muscles are torn, the body replaces a rather neat, organized network of a combination of yellow elastic, and dense white non-elastic collagen fibers, with a rather haphazard array of dense white connective scar tissue. This scar tissue will help hold bones together (aka: Joints) but doesn't have the same type and combination of strength and resiliency that the original connective tissue had. At the junction of the original tissue and the new scar tissue is a transitional zone

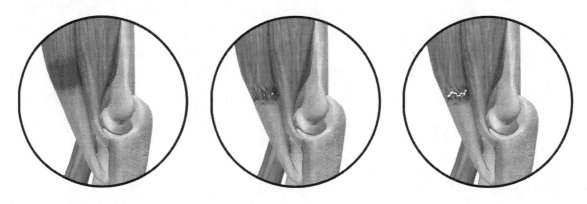

Illustration 18, Three degrees of sprains or strains

that is more prone to tearing & re-injury as are most transitional zones in the body. The new scar tissue being less resilient causes a loss of range of motion at the joint level of the injury and therefore increases the stress upon that joint due to reduced and altered biomechanical function. Loss of range of motion also causes aberrant afferent input into the nervous system which can become painful as well." (21)

The above illustrations are reflective of the tearing to soft tissue our clients present to us daily.

Imagine a textbook or encyclopedia with thousands of these pictures.

Therefore I say, almost every pain we address is about tearing soft tissue.

Before I present a formula for addressing specific soft tissue complaints, we need to review our trigger point approach.

Do You Remember Your Trigger Point Training?

If there was a bible or holy grail for massage therapists it would be Myofascial Pain and Dysfunction, The Trigger Point Manual by Drs. Janet Travell and David Simons.

These two amazing physicians spent their entire lives studying and effectively addressing and eliminating pain.

Their two part textbook on addressing soft tissue pain, in my opinion, changed our world.

Even though Travell and Simons laid down the foundations of working with pain by providing us the road map for addressing trigger points it was one of their disciples and patients, fitness phenom Bonnie Prudden that taught us how to use our hands in administering trigger point therapy.

Remember, both Travell and Simons were medical doctors.

They mapped out the trigger points, but a major part of their treatment protocol used injections.

For all intents and purposes, it was Bonnie Prudden that invented or more accurately re-discovered the trigger point therapy system massage therapists use today.

I say re-discovered because Osteopath's having been doing this sophisticated type of work since the early 1900's.

Bonnie's pain erasure formula instructed us to identify the painful area, map out the trigger points, compress and hold each specific point and then stretch out the area.

Bonnie is in my opinion, the Godmother of modern day medical massage.

Here's what Wikipedia has to say about Bonnie's discovery of holding points to address soft tissue pain.

"In January 1969 at age 55, Prudden put in a call to Travell. In March of that year she began regular monthly trips to Travell's office in Washington, DC receiving a series of trigger point injections designed to make her more comfortable and save her hip. During the summer of 1970 she had her right hip replaced. It was 1976 before all the pieces of the myotherapy puzzle fell into place. Prudden's working arrangement with Dr. Desmond Tivy, M.D. was that he would send the patient to Prudden who would find the trigger points, mark them and send them back to Dr. Tivy who would inject. The patient would them come back to Prudden for the corrective exercises. One morning a woman arrived with her head lopsided and with a stiff and painful neck. Later Prudden would say that she may have pressed the trigger point a little longer or pressed it harder when she was marking the point. However, afterward the woman no longer had pain, or a stiff neck and her head was straight. So began her development of Bonnie Prudden Myotherapy. Over the next four years using herself as a

guinea pig, experimenting with staff, friends and patients she developed and mapped out the most common trigger points and the accompanying corrective exercises. It was Dr. Tivy who coined the word MYOTHERAPY and said that there were not many modalities available to him such as this with few side effects." (22) (23)

Another word about this great, amazing woman, Bonnie Prudden.

"In 1955, armed with statistics and a personal invitation to the Eisenhower White House, Bonnie Prudden presented her findings on the fitness level of American public-school children compared to that of their peers in Europe. This became known as The Report that Shocked the President or the Shape of the Nation and was the beginning of a change in American attitudes toward physical fitness." (24)

> *Trigger point work is one of the few natural options soft tissue specialists have to address pain.*

You might remember the President's Commission on Physical Fitness from gym class in public school.

That's when every student had to do specific exercises and be tested in things like squat thrusts, chin ups and running all different distances.

It was Bonnie Prudden that was the co-founder of that Commission, originally called the President's Council on Youth Fitness.

Did you ever see the trigger point charts you can put on your wall?

I have a set of them and at some time during my career referred to them regularly.

At this time in my career, any point that is sensitive I treat as if it is a trigger point.

Here's what I do.

I hold all points (even shiatsu points) for a minimum of 8 seconds or longer.

Whenever you hold (compress) a point, after 8 seconds of being deprived of oxygen and blood flow, the nerve begins to shut down and the muscle will begin to un-splint and relax.

If there is pain it will begin to subside.

As soon as you release the pressure, with the re-emergence of blood and oxygen, the nerve will kick back on, pushing the muscle back into pain and spasm.

It will not go back 100% though. Each time you hold the trigger point, the muscle will lessen the splinting and pain.

Over a period of time and sessions, the muscles will go back to be a happy family.

Trigger point work is one of the few natural options soft tissue specialists have to address pain.

In 1985, at the American Massage Therapy National Convention in Seattle, Washington, I took a trigger point class with the founder of the Chicago School of Massage, the late Bob King.

You might recall, Bob was also the American Massage therapy Association's National President.

Bob said his highly successful **treatment secret** was to apply hydroculator steam packs after clearing the trigger points and stretching out the patient.

The hot packs, he said would increase circulation and lessen the possibility of pain afterwards.

The rule is, anything that increases circulation will speed healing, decrease pain and spasm and very often lessen sensitivity the day after.

The rule is, anything that increases circulation will speed healing, decrease pain and spasm and very often lessen sensitivity the day after.

In those days, a hydroculator was kind of pricey, costing over $600. Now it's under $300.

I bought one none the less and found it to be an extraordinary improvement to my practice.

Something other soft tissue therapist like physical therapists and chiropractors have known forever.

I now have hydroculators in every treatment room.

I believe the combination of trigger point work, stretching and hot packs was and still is a game-changer for my career as a massage therapist.

How to address a specific soft tissue complaint

I am an old school massage therapist.

Before we had our present license, massage therapists were told that they were not allowed to treat any specific soft tissue conditions.

We gave a good, relaxing rub but when it came to folks wondering if we could help them with a specific complaint, like back pain, it was illegal to say we did. Only doctors and their physical therapists were legal. Two things came of that issue. One is that we had to answer the questions very carefully and two, we had to be able to treat every trigger point, every tear, every pain within the scope of our massage. So, I created a massage session that would clear trigger points and address tears and imbalances without the diagnostic luxuries of today like simple muscle testing.

At my school, we taught a class called scripts. It was dedicated to answering each question legally but not to put ourselves in jeopardy or out of business. We learned how to address problem areas without diagnostic assessment and to treat a complaint without saying we could.

Sixty-five thousand massages later…

I have a specific protocol for addressing complaints.

It's my go to formula when I do not have a clear picture of the situation even after reading the intake and then interviewing my client.

My client says he overstretched his shoulder in yoga class a week ago.

He iced it initially when he got home from class and in the days following he used heat and a topical to lessen the discomfort.

By the end of the week he decided to come in for a massage session.

His opening statement to me was, "I think I have a frozen shoulder."

When I tested the shoulders mobility, it was indeed quite limited and with minimal range of motion displayed great tenderness.

The entire musculature of the shoulder was in spasm.

Soft tissue therapy guru, Erik Dalton says, *"Protective spasm is the brain's reflexogenic attempt to prevent further insult to injured tissues. By splinting the area with spasm, muscle 'locking' effectively reduces painful joint movements."* (24)

When I think of a frozen shoulder, I generally think of rotator cuff involvement.

Specifically subscapularis, but without a medical assessment or an MRI, how do I really know.

The new generation of massage therapists are savvier than I when it comes to assessment.

Massage therapy has come a long way and eventually to become an LMT you will have to go to university for five years like they did in the former Soviet Union.

For my frozen shoulder guy, I could refer out at this point but my client was dead set against that idea.

"This is just a simple strain Larry, I am not going to an ortho guy where he will take six months off my life with his God damn x-ray machine!"

True story.

So here's what I do and did.

One of my rules is to cause no pain.

I tell students to address the musculature as if you were peeling an onion one layer at a time.

A good massage therapist prepares the musculature by gradually desensitizing a region.

When asked by students how deeply to we go in? Five pounds of pressure, ten pounds, twenty pounds?

Cause no pain.

My answer has always been starting at the *"point of resistance."*

When you begin to apply pressure on a specific spot, go in very tentatively until the soft tissue resists any more pressure.

That is the point of resistance.

Imagine a client coming to you and saying, *"I hate deep tissue work. I do not want any pain. Please just a light relaxing massage."*

If you start at the point of resistance, the soft tissue will desensitize, and you can very gingerly go from there.

Over a period of time, that client will acclimate to your touch and might begin to enjoy a deeper massage experience.

It won't feel deeper to them because you gradually desensitized the region.

Once used to deeper work and possibly more therapeutic work, they will never go back to the light stuff again.

Now you have a lifetime commitment.

Now back to my clients alleged frozen shoulder.

Here's what I did.

I warmed up the muscles in the upper back, neck and shoulders with simple effleurage and then petrissage.

Light palpation to discern what's going on.

I slowly stretch and strip the muscles with a very light touch.

Stretch and strip is a technique I teach all the time.

By putting a muscle into mild extension, I can strip down the superficial fascia with a forearm, thumb or hand.

Then I began holding points with thumb compression.

It takes 8 seconds of pressure to begin the process of turning off the pain. It happens by depriving the nerve of oxygen and blood flow.

I always ask my client to tell me any points that might be sensitive.

You know they rarely ever do, but I'm looking for any sign of sensitivity.

A blink of an eyelash, a movement of a finger or toe. Any indication of sensitivity whatsoever. If they give me one, I'll gently ask, *"Was that area a little sensitive?"*

If the answer is yes, I will lighten my pressure and extend my eight second holding pattern to thirty seconds.

If the pain is substantial, I might hold the point for as much as a minute or even two.

Sometimes trigger points try to get away, so I'll clear the points a quarter inch above, a quarter inch below, to the left and to the right.

I call that a *"round robin."*

After turning off the trigger points in the region, the muscles should be a little happier with much less spasm.

It's then that I'll look for the source and origin of our pain.

Again simply by palpating, holding points and looking for positive feedback.

In this case, the culprit was an injury to the anterior deltoid and not the subscap.

Upon further palpation, I found the exact spot.

It announced itself with a scream from my client along with his eyes seemingly bugging out of his head.

That's when I performed some simple cross fiber friction, Dr. Cyriax style.

Dr. Cyriax is considered by many to be the Father of Orthopedic Medicine. *(2)

The technique he popularized is deep, transverse friction to the soft tissue.

Applying deep friction across the grain of the muscles, break up adhesions, scar tissue, increases blood flow and dramatically speeds up healing.

Dr. Cyriax taught us to start very lightly and very gradually go deeper.

A cross fiber session was to be done daily for 8 to 12 minutes.

Since it's not realistic to assume our client will be coming in everyday, odds are you will have to teach the cross-fiber technique to your client for their own self-care.

Immediately after my cross-fiber treatment, I apply hydroculator hot packs.

Like I said earlier, this increases circulation and whenever you increase circulation you decrease pain and speed healing.

That's why ice works, heat works, ultrasound, even magnets.

I concluded the session with simple stretching.

I usually explain to my clients that nothing happens overnight and it usually takes multiple sessions to correct something that hurts so much.

They will feel a bit better after the session but very often, by the evening or next day the pain can come back with a vengeance.

After all trigger point work with stretching and cross fiber can be invasive even when you have a gentle touch.

Imagine us taking an exercise class. It is quite normal to get charley horse the day after a good workout.

I always have this vision that my client is at home later that evening, perhaps watching television and that spot begins to act up again.

I can see them turning to their significant other and saying, *"How do you like that guy, I went to him for relief. I'm worse now than I was before!*

But he did say this might happen, so I'm going to give him the benefit of the doubt and continue with my treatments."

All in all it took four sessions to correct my client's issue.

Soft Tissue Protocol

Whenever a client comes in for a session, I'll ask do you have any pain or specific areas that need attention.

Very often they will say, *"I strained my back,"* or *"I sprained something somewhere."*

When I tell them the definition of a sprain or strain, they'll say, "Well Larry, I don't really think I tore something. Maybe I just pulled the muscle playing soccer."

I'll explain to them a muscle strain or a pulled muscle is easy to do. All that's required to tear is to over-extend.

Something as simple as picking up a pen from the floor can result in a tear to a hamstring.

Just about every injury a soft tissue therapist address is about over-extending or tearing.

The rule is every time you ask a prospective client where it hurts, consider you are addressing torn and damaged muscle tissue.

Here's my general massage therapy protocol:

Warm-up muscles.

Stretch and strip area in question

Clear all trigger points in region.

Identify troubled spot with palpation. The spot should announce itself.

Cross fiber friction for 8-12 minutes starting very lightly and gradually increasing pressure.

Apply heat to prevent bruising.

Stretch region.

Repeat as necessary.

THE PARADIGM SHIFT: Here it is!

How to Assess What Is Weakening the Soft Tissue

Remember our chart from earlier

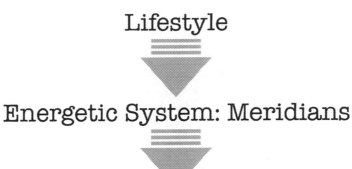

Lifestyle

Energetic System: Meridians

Soft Tissue

Skeletal Structure

Lifestyle directly affects the internal organs and their energy lines (the meridians) especially when you consume more than the organs can handle.

The energy lines (the meridians) are direct extensions of the internal organs.

So, for all intents and purposes they are part of the internal organs.

They run throughout the body.

When the lifestyle is in balance, the meridians are strong and healthy and therein the soft tissue functions optimally.

The body, mind and spirit are healthy.

When the lifestyle is in excess, those specific excessive organs/meridians are weak and imbalanced and therein the soft tissue is compromised.

Weaker, injury prone, making it easier to get injured, soft tissue wise.

So that brings us to the last discussion, our lifestyle.

According to all my amazing teachers and a personal lifetime of study and practice, it's our lifestyle choices that determines almost everything.

I say almost everything because there are aspects that we can't control, like genetics, environmental exposures, accidents, etc.

I'm talking about what you put into your mouth and head.

There is no separation between body, mind, emotions or spirit in Oriental medicine.

If there is an organ that is out of balance, it will affect other aspects of who you are.

So a compromised liver per se will affect how you feel, even how you think.

Chinese medicine has studied this for five thousand years.

Imagine if you will:

You've been getting bottled up lately, anxious, impatient, even angry at times.

You tail the guy in the left lane if they are going to slow.

You're jumping down the kid's throats, and you have no patience for the stupidity of the human race.

In fact, the more you hang with humans, the more you long for being home with your dog or cats.

You go to the doctor and tell her about your short fuse.

Doc says one of the following:

1. I'm going to write you a script for a mild anti-depressant, just temporarily, just to get you over the hump at this time in your life.

No meat, no dairy, no sugar, no simple carbs, three weeks, no anger!

2. I'm going to write you a script for an anti-anxiety med, just to even you out for when you need it.

3. I'm going to send you to our group's psychiatrist, just to get a work-up, to make sure everything's ok.

4. I'm going to refer you to a licensed professional counselor, so you can develop some positive strategies on how not to give up your power when people press your buttons.

While that last one would be great for anyone, if you went to one of my teachers, they would say the following:

"No meat, no dairy, no sugar, no simple carbs, three weeks, no anger!"

The word for anger in Japanese is "kan shaku," which translates, "liver illness."

That's the reason the French say when you are angry, "Don't get your Gaul up!"

In Oriental medicine, there is no separation between the body and your emotions.

If one is compromised, they both are.

When an organ is over-worked, it has a direct affect/effect on your body, mind, emotions and spirit.

The Chinese say, from the one great spirit, come the two opposing forces.

In other words, from the one absolute energy, come yin and yang, male and female, infra-red and ultra-violet, black and white, hot and cold, alpha and omega.

Yin and yang are constantly seeking each other out to create greater balance.

Just like electrons in the Periodic Chart of Elements looking to balance the electrons in their outer shells.

The Gospel of Thomas (50), translated by Stephen Patterson and Marvin Meyer, Jesus said, *"If they ask you, 'What is the evidence of your Father in you?' say to them, 'It is motion and a rest.'"*

In ancient times, the Chinese believed that God showed him/herself in every aspect of life.

It's part of their Cosmology, their understanding of the universe.

This yin/yang concept is the basis of Asian theories of health, medicine, and philosophy.

For thousands of years they observed the Tao (pronounced Dow, meaning the Way), defined as the study on how nature presents itself.

Its natural laws, its obvious displays, like everything green in Springtime.

If they could live in alignment, harmoniously in balance with the Way of things (Tao), they felt they were living within God's law.

That's why they called in Taoism and make that black and white yin/yang sign.

So that brings us to the yin and yang of the human body.

When it comes to the organs of the human body, this is how they are married: they are presented yang first, yin second.

There are twelve meridians, ten organ, two functions.

For clarity sake, the two functions are the heart governor, sometimes referred to as the pericardium and the triple warmer or heater. The heart governor is associated with the circulatory system and the triple heater is the body heating and cooling system and thermostat.

Fire Element	Heart/Small Intestines
	Heart Governor/Triple Warmer
Earth Element	Spleen/Stomach
Metal Element	Lungs/Large Intestine
Water Element	kidneys/Bladder
Wood Element	Liver/Gall Bladder

And like any relationship, if something happens to your significant other it will affect you as well.

One spouse is there for the other.

It's the same for the internal organs: since kidneys and bladder are married, if something happens to the kidneys, it will affect the bladder, and vice versa.

So Chinese doctors look at the married organ pairs together. When doing your massage, it is helpful to familiarize yourself with the acupuncture meridian lines and while learning them to have a chart available to use as a reference guide. The large intestine lines (meridians) for instance are on both sides of the body and many points (tsubos) can be used to assess the large intestines condition. For the large intestine alone, you can find these points on the hands, shoulders, ears, abs, along the spine, the back, even on the bottom of the feet. So, in effect, it's like a system wide assessment. A practitioner that is familiar with the meridians can discern whether a sensitive point indicates a localized problem around the site or a system wide imbalance indicating an organ condition. When the large intestine is compromised, maybe say from a chronic lack of fiber, its meridian lines will be imbalanced.

The areas associated with the organs are usually directly over the internal organ itself and then along its meridian line.

The large intestine lines run through the shoulders, so shoulder issues bring that organ to mind; weight training, holding your tension there, keyboarding for long periods of time on the computer, putting the phone between the ear and shoulder for hands free talking, to name some. My teachers however would say one of the main contributing causes of tight, stiff shoulders is a chronic lack of fiber.

Let's see how it all lays out.

Some guidelines:

Excess nutrition shows up as a detox over the internal organ or its meridian line: Whether you bounce your legs, sneeze, cough, excessively blink, sweat, get eczema, pimples, talk to loudly, have cold or hot hands, a red complexion, the list is endless, all of these are discharges of excess. It's all the excess leaving the body that we're looking at. That's the concentrate concept. When you're eating high up on the food chain, you discharge constantly and age much more quickly.

The areas associated with the organs are usually directly over the internal organ itself and then along its meridian line. Wherever the pain, hardness or irregularity is located, first think, what internal organ is just below. Is it possible there might be a relationship? Especially if it's an organ that has been pounded by poor nutritional choices. Next, remembering the meridian is an extension of the internal organ, what meridian is the irregularity or imbalance coming out on?

Is it possible there might be a relationship? Finally, there are other relationships that are to be considered as well. Louise Hay in her NY Times best-selling book, Heal Your Body: The Mental Causes for Physical Illness and the Metaphysical Way To Overcome Them, shares her insights on the emotional connections of our physical complaints. Some of my teachers even talk about the growing patterns of the embryo in utero. For example, the small intestine and the brain grow at the exact same time, even look alike, therefore believed to have a connection, a symbiosis. This type of thinking is the basis for other diagnostic arts such as reflexology, zone therapy, and the Japanese system of Karenbui.

The signs of organ imbalance have been gathered over thousands of years and is the basis of traditional Oriental medicine.

The Chinese Clock is part of the Five-element theory, a study. Essentially it indicates the timing of the high and low energy patterns for each organ and meridian. When someone tells you that they have a specific complaint that has a time associated with it, think Chinese Clock. For instance, an insomnia complaint. What time do you wake up every night? If they tell you there is a regular time pattern, look up the time the organ it is related to. Let's say you go to bed every evening at ten o'clock and you find a disturbed sleep pattern that wakes you every night at 1:30 AM. When you look up what organ is at its peak energy level at 1:30 AM, you'll discover that is liver time. Knowing that can help you modify your lifestyle to address the liver imbalance. Maybe you eliminate fat consumption at the dinner meal or cut down your fat consumption generally. Perhaps you start taking liver support products like alpha lipoic acid, lemon water or a liver flush.

Associated emotions connect the organ imbalance with the entire body-mind connection. There is no separation, if you have an organ imbalance it will affect every other part of your life; the way you think, feel, move, look, express yourself, etc.

The Elements

Fire Element

Heart, Small Intestine, Heart Governor, Triple Warmer

Food that influence organs/meridians: fruit sugar, fruit juice, hot spices, out of season foods, dead, lifeless food (distilled or reverse osmosis water), irradiated food, coffee, heavy aromatics (strong herbs), excess spicy foods, chocolate, sugar, salt, vinegar, garlic, alcohol, genetically modified foods with pesticides and herbicides attack intestinal flora, meat, cheese.

Areas associated with Heart/Small Intestines and Heart Governor/Triple Warmer:

Edema, swelling, hardness, discoloration, temperature changes and abnormalities along the meridians.

- **The heart meridians (9 tsubos)** are in the center of the chest and back, runs through the diaphragm down into the small intestine. On the extremity the meridian runs through the lung and down the inside of the arm to the inside little pinky.
- **The small intestine meridians (19 tsubos)** run from the pinky finger up the outside of the forearm, over the elbow, to the back of the shoulder at the upper back/base of the neck. It then crosses the neck, cheek, outer corner of the eye and ends at the ear.
- **The heart governor meridians (9 tsubos)** begin in the chest at the double walled protecting sac called the pericardium. An outlet travels down the diaphragm to the three areas of the triple warmer. Another outlet of the main channel crosses over and appears outside the nipple, travels briefly up around the armpit then travels down the inside arm (biceps and biceps tendon at elbow crease), then down the center of he flexors, mid hand to the outer corner of the middle finger.
- **The triple warmer meridians** (thorax, abdomen, and pelvis) originate from the outside tip of the ring finger, through the space between the ring and pinky fingers, on to the wrist, up the extensors, through the tip of the elbow, and up the back of the arm to the shoulder. It connects at the chest with the pericardium innervating the upper, middle and lower burners and eventually at the collarbone, the side of the neck and around the back of the ear.

Heart Meridian

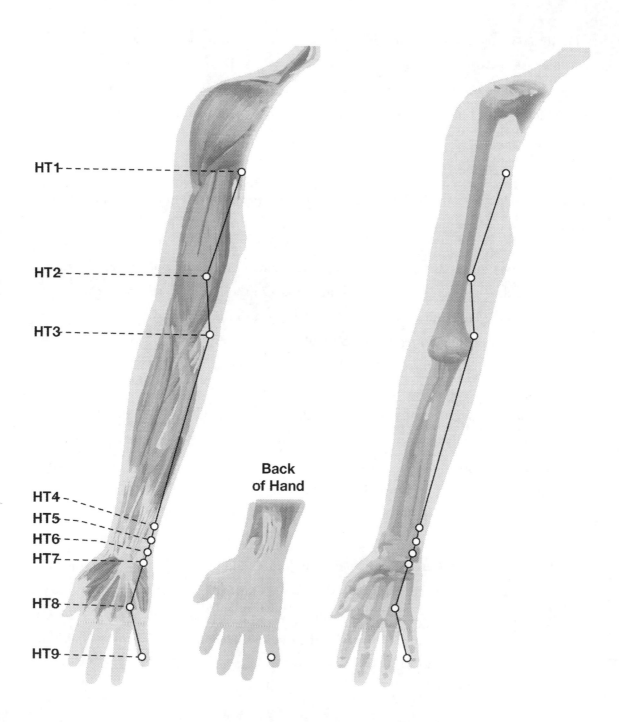

HT1

HT2

HT3

Back of Hand

HT4
HT5
HT6
HT7

HT8

HT9

Illustration 19

Small Intestine Meridian
(Arm and Back)

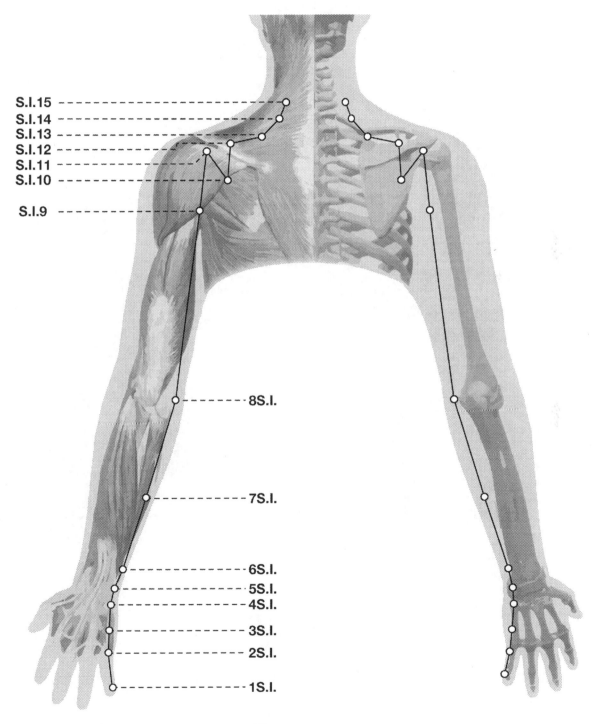

S.I.15
S.I.14
S.I.13
S.I.12
S.I.11
S.I.10

S.I.9

8S.I.

7S.I.

6S.I.
5S.I.
4S.I.

3S.I.

2S.I.

1S.I.

Illustration 20

Small Intestine Meridian
(Head)

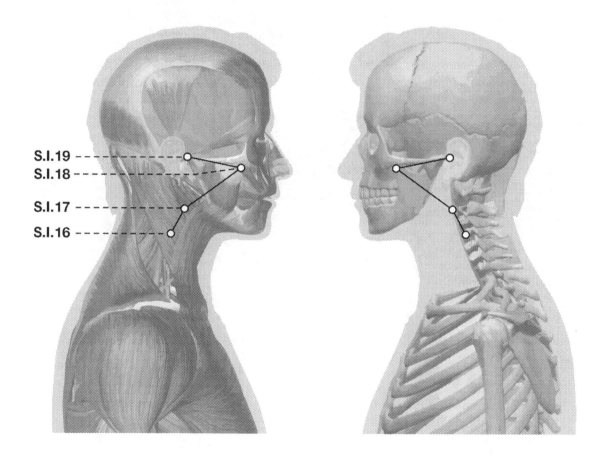

S.I.19
S.I.18
S.I.17
S.I.16

Illustration 21

Heart Governor

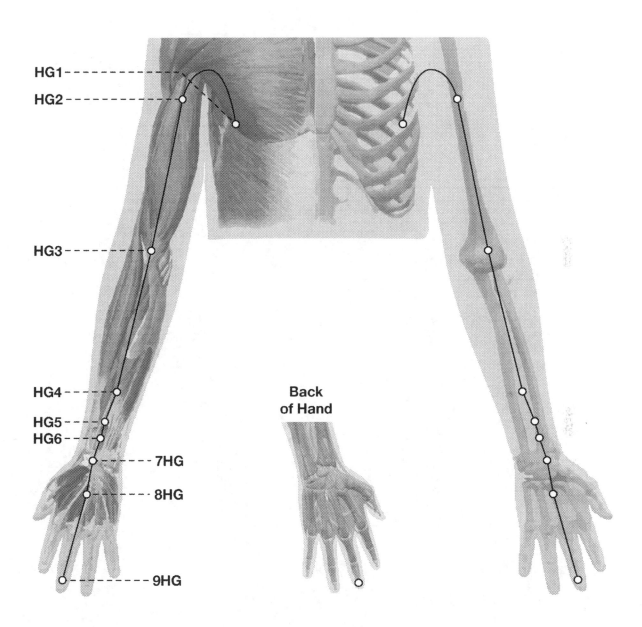

HG1
HG2

HG3

HG4

HG5
HG6

7HG

8HG

Back of Hand

9HG

Illustration 22

73

Triple Warmer Meridian
(Arms)

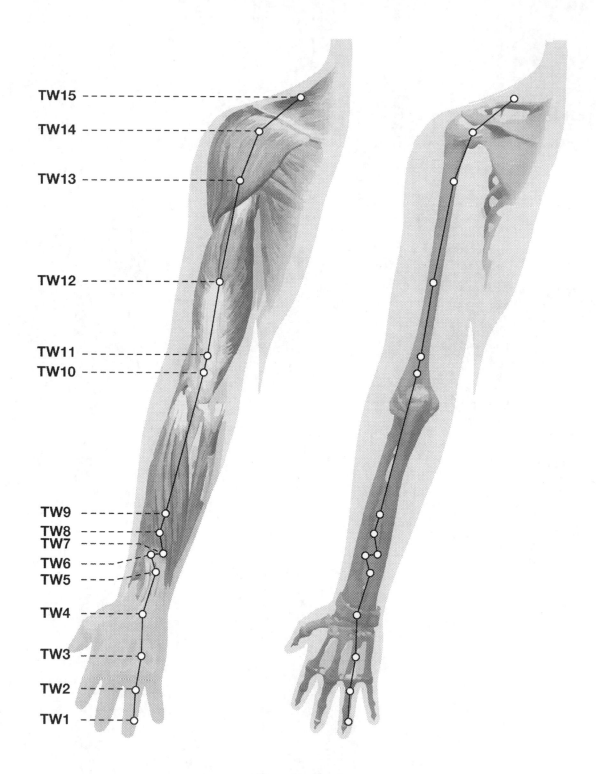

TW15
TW14
TW13
TW12
TW11
TW10
TW9
TW8
TW7
TW6
TW5
TW4
TW3
TW2
TW1

Illustration 23

Triple Warmer Meridian

(Head)

TW23 - - - - - - - - -
TW22 - - - - - - - - -
TW21 - - - - - - - - -
TW20 - - - - - - - - -
TW19 - - - - - - - - -
TW18 - - - - - - - - -
TW17 - - - - - - - - -
TW16 - - - - - - - - -

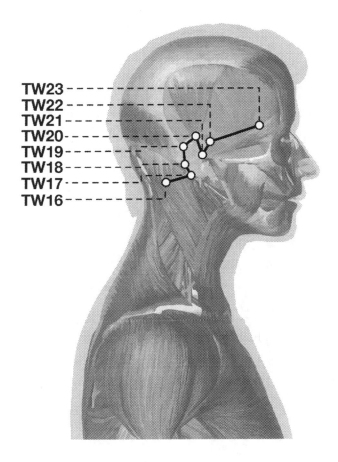
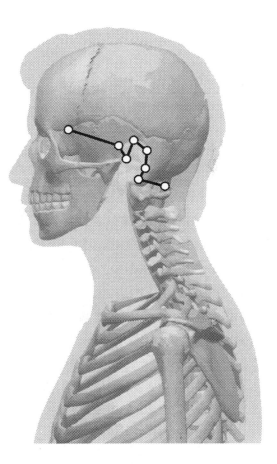

Illustration 24

Signs of Imbalance: heart controls how you speak and speech problems, talking incessantly, tip of tongue redness, red face, swollen puffy red face, swollen nose, hands show the condition of the heart, reddish or hot hands indicate heart over working or blood pressure condition, wet hands indicates excess consumption of liquid, excessive strong grip heart overworking or high blood pressure, weak grip equals deficient heart energy, lack of mental clarity, scattered energy finds it difficult to focus.

Time of Day (Chinese Clock): The hours for heart, 11am to 1pm, hours for small intestine, 1pm to 3pm. The hours for the Heart governor are 7pm-9pm, the hours for the triple warmer is 9pm-11pm.

Emotions: agitation, insomnia and palpitations, joy, excitement, heartache, sadness, love for self and others, hysteria, hypersensitivity, prejudice and hatred (hardening of arteries)

Notes: We must consider what happens to our body when we eat non-local foods, or out-of-season foods. Non-local foods are foods that grow in tropical climates like chocolate, coffee, sugar, mango, pineapple, orange juice, and especially hot spices. In every hot climate, they eat hot spices to cool themselves off, like Mexico, Vietnam, Indonesia, and Thailand. If it's 110 degrees in India, and you don't eat the hot spices, like the curry, it's almost unbearable. That's the way nature works. It provides you what you need for the region you are living in. It's the same for all tropical countries where the food is very spicy, sweet, juicy, fragrant and cooling.

But none of these tropical foods grow here in the northeast where I reside. They are imported to us. They are not native to our region. The weather here is temperate and chillier three seasons out of four. If you eat the tropical diet in a temperate zone, my teachers say your nervous system will break down and when you get old, you'll begin to shake not to mention being cold all the time. Non-seasonal foods are foods eaten during a season when they are not normally flourishing. For example, eating watermelon, tomatoes, cucumbers or spinach in the winter. When the summertime is here, all those wonderful fruits and vegetables are growing. At the first frost, many summertime vegetables and fruits will die off. The things that are hearty and strong enough to handle the weather changing are acorn squash, butternut squash, parsnips, onions, brussel sprouts, kale, carrots—all are hearty enough to handle the cold weather. If you stop eating the foods that die immediately, and you start eating the veggies that can handle the frost, then you can handle the frost more easily, and your body will be warmer in winter as opposed to colder. You'll be eating in accord with your geography. That makes a big difference to your heart/small intestine, heart governor/triple warmer.

A word about concentrates and how they age your body and directly affect your Energetic System:

"Concentrates" are foods that are very high up on the food chain. When we're eating high up on the food chain, there's more that needs to be burned.

Animal flesh is the big one. That animal has to eat a lot of grain to make the flesh we eat. So indirectly when we eat the animal, we are eating all the grains it consumed along the way. A chicken has to eat a pound of grain for each egg it lays. So if we go to the diner and get a spinach omelet, it might contain 4 or 5 eggs, which is the equivalent of 4 or 5 pounds of grain that you just ate for breakfast. That's enough grain like brown rice and lentils, to feed you healthy for a couple of days. You just ate a couple days' worth of food for breakfast. Then we go over to Joey's house to watch the football game. He brings out a big bucket of fried chicken. If you're sitting around drinking beer, it's easy to eat a lot of that chicken. A pound of chicken is around 3 or 4 pounds of feed. So that chicken has to eat 4 pounds of grain to make one pound of its flesh. And you can eat a pound of chicken in one sitting. So you just consumed the equivalent of 4 pounds of grain for breakfast and another 4 pounds for lunch. Since our team won, we decide to celebrate by going to the steak house. That one-pound sirloin sounds really good, so you order "the belly buster." It takes 13 pounds of grain to produce one pound of beef. Really high up on the food chain. Thirteen pounds is enough to feed one-person sufficient food to last almost two weeks! All in all, you ate the equivalent of 21 pounds of grains in one day. When we eat way, way high up on the food chain like this, we overwhelm our internal organs with the excess, our body ages and wears out much faster, eventually creating serious imbalances throughout your entire system.

Flesh foods are not the only concentrates.

Sugar is also a concentrate. It takes ten pounds of sugar cane to make one pound of sugar. A can of cola soda contains 10 teaspoons of sugar. A slice of chocolate cake contains 6 to 12 teaspoons.

There are also other concentrates. Let's say we go out for a brunch. The waitress says that they have fresh squeezed Florida orange juice, and since she made it sound so attractive, I have some. A glass of orange juice is the sugar of four oranges. Now we would not have four oranges at one meal, but you just drank the sugar of four oranges. If you're on weight watchers, you're allowed to have 2 ounces of juice, that's the equivalent of one fruit. While I'm getting food from the buffet, the waitress refills the glass. I feel obligated to drink it since there are starving children in India, but I don't want to because it's way too much sugar, now eight oranges. A glass of apple juice is 6 teaspoons of sugar; apple cider is 8 teaspoons; a quarter-cup of raisins is 4 teaspoons of sugar.

Earth Element

Spleen and Stomach

Food that influences organ/meridians: sugars, simple carbs, foods with a high glycemic index (flour products, potatoes, sugars)

Areas associated with Spleen/Stomach: Edema, swelling, hardness, discoloration, temperature changes and abnormalities along spleen/stomach meridians

- **The spleen meridians (18 tsubos)** start at the outside tip of the big toe and runs up the inside of the calf (tibialis anterior), thigh (adductors), up the suspender route around the outer chest by the nipple to the collarbone and lats.

- **The stomach meridians (45 tsubos)** start just under the eye, to the cheek bone then outside of the lip. It curves up to the forehead and then turns back to the shoulder, ribs, in a straight line along the stomach, and then down the leg ending at the outside of the second toe.

Signs of Imbalance: if big toe curves toward second toe, bunions on outside of big toe, rhomboids on the left side just over spleen/stomach organs, bloating, stomach swelling, blood sugar imbalances, poor appetite, tiredness after eating, lack of energy, cracked heels, dry and cracked lips, excessive thirst, provides nutrients for muscle and energy metabolism (when spleen/stomach is diseased muscle will be atrophied and show abnormal physical weakness), sores around mouth, tension in jaw, abdominal pain, intestinal upset, constipation, infertility related to endometriosis/uterine fibroids/ heavy periods, need for stimulants (tobacco, caffeine, cravings for carbohydrates), breast problems, breast sensitivity towards the armpits (lumps/cysts/sensitivity prior to menstruation or ovulation), low energy levels, thyroid problems, weight problems (being overweight or underweight), when people eat a lot of sugar, they excessively blink all the time.

Time of Day (Chinese Clock): The hours for stomach are 7-9am, the hours for the spleen are 9-11am

Associated Emotion: worry, indecision, skepticism, dwelling or focusing too much on a particular topic, anxiety, doubt, jealousy, over thinking.

Spleen Meridian
(Legs)

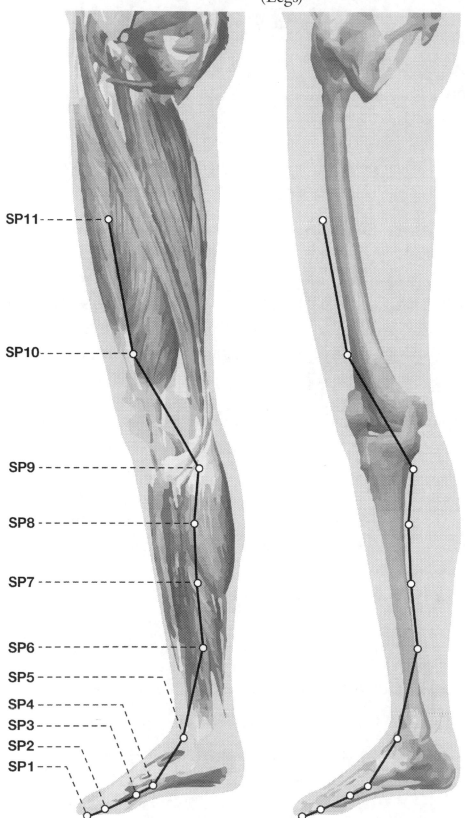

SP11
SP10
SP9
SP8
SP7
SP6
SP5
SP4
SP3
SP2
SP1

Illustration 25

Spleen Meridian

(Torso)

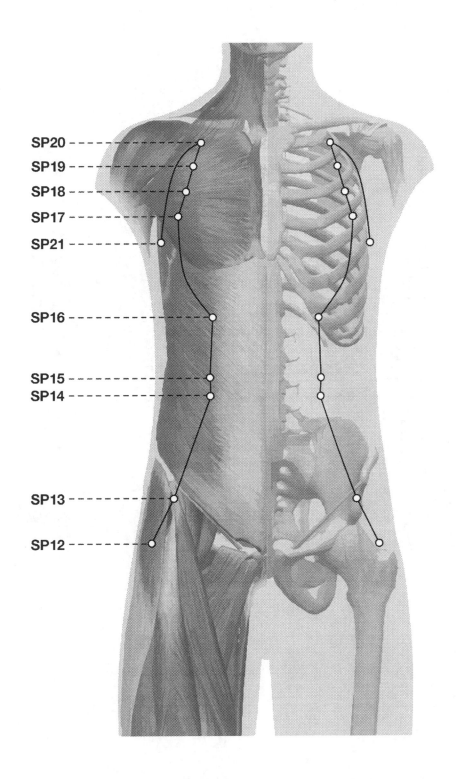

SP20
SP19
SP18
SP17
SP21
SP16
SP15
SP14
SP13
SP12

Illustration 26

Stomach Meridian

(Head)

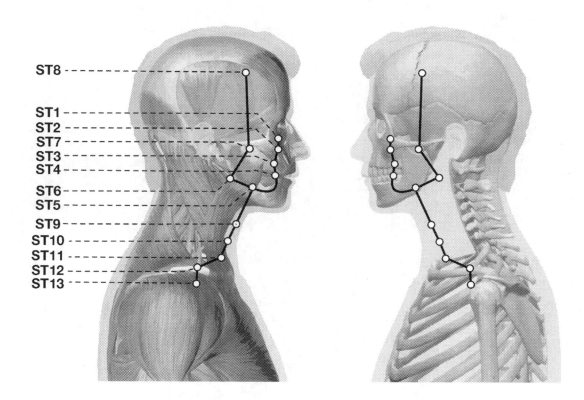

ST8
ST1
ST2
ST7
ST3
ST4
ST6
ST5
ST9
ST10
ST11
ST12
ST13

Illustration 27

Stomach Meridian
(Torso)

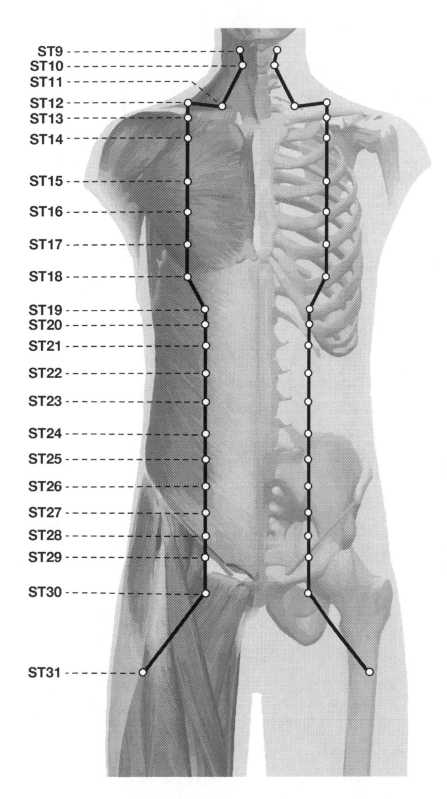

ST9
ST10
ST11
ST12
ST13
ST14
ST15
ST16
ST17
ST18
ST19
ST20
ST21
ST22
ST23
ST24
ST25
ST26
ST27
ST28
ST29
ST30
ST31

Illustration 28

Stomach Meridian
(Legs)

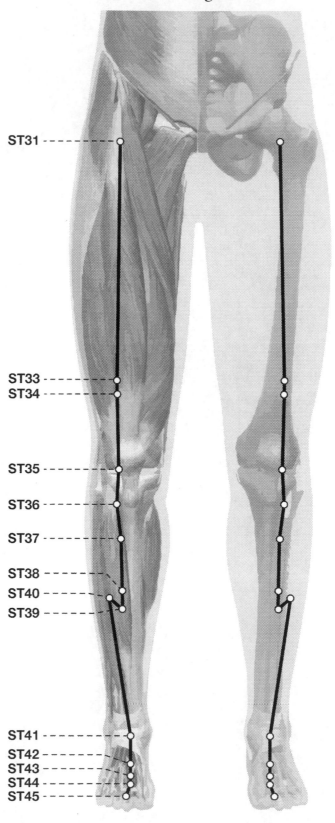

ST31

ST33
ST34

ST35

ST36

ST37

ST38
ST40
ST39

ST41
ST42
ST43
ST44
ST45

Illustration 29

Notes: Foods with a high Glycemic Index (e.g. white bread, table sugar, white potato, white rice) cause your blood sugar to spike quickly. When it comes to sugars, the simple sugars and simple carbs are going to affect you the most. Once we developed the glycemic index, we started realizing that not all flour products are the same. Traditionally, if you were diagnosed with diabetes, the dietician would take you off pasta. Then they found that certain pastas, those made with hard winter wheat, were ok to eat because they have a low glycemic index. We usually don't eat foods singularly, but in combinations, where the glycemic index is different. The pasta I get is called Bio-Nature; it is a mainstream brand made of hard winter wheat that comes from Italy, it's organic, and sold at all the health food stores and in many supermarkets, now. It has no fiber because it's white flour, but it has a low glycemic index, so it doesn't turn quickly to sugar. Let's say you mix that with greens and beans; you'd get your fiber in the beans and kale, and you don't have to worry about the lack of fiber in the winter wheat because everything will move though.

As to the emotions that are associated with the spleen and stomach (indecision and skepticism), I recall Michio Kushi was teaching the class and talked about the range of emotional symptoms associated with blood sugar. You'll always know when a person has spleen or stomach problem because they have a sing song voice said Kushi. To make the point he illustrated the vocal sound and an individual with an imbalanced spleen might make, *"Helloooo, how you doeeeeng? I can't believe it's you-oooo!"* Their voice will go up and down, sing-song. Kushi continued, folks with sugar imbalances tend to be indecisive and skeptical.

"Would you like to eat Italian food tonight or Indian food?" "Uh, I don't know, whatever you like."
In that same class earlier, a guy got up to go to the lavatory. Kushi, a master of Oriental diagnosis, paused the class to make his point and said, the fella that just went to the men's room, I have never met before, but I can tell you from observation, he has a blood sugar disorder. Kushi then briefly talked about the emotional and physical symptoms a person with sugar problems might display. When the guy came back, Kushi addressed him directly, "Let me ask you, sir, what do you think of this class so far?" The guy responded in a sing song voice, "Well with all due respect, Mr. Kushi, I'm kind of skeptical about the things you are talking about today." At that point the whole class erupted. Kushi then asked him what he was there for, and the gentleman replied, "I've been having blood sugar problems that I'm afraid is going to turn into diabetes at some point. Diabetes runs in my family. I was going back and forth about where I should go and whom I should work with and my friends strongly encouraged me to take your program. I think I waited too long though, I should have come years ago when my condition was just in the beginning stages. And that's exactly what Kushi had said he was gonna say—he nailed it. We see this all the time.

An interesting aside: When I was in my early twenties at my first Kushi class, Sensei was teaching us the pressure points to assess and diagnose particular organ conditions of the body. Spleen 10 is just above the inside of the knee on the thigh, and when you press this point, if you're a sugar person, this point will light up and hurt like the dickens. I had my legs crossed over each other, and Kushi comes over and puts a good grip on my Spleen 10 point—I yelled and leaped up. The whole class looks up from their pressure point practice and Kushi looks at me with a big grin and says, *"No hope for you."*

Everyone cracked up laughing and that simple intervention of hitting my sugar point changed the way I ate forever!

Metal Element

Lungs and Large Intestine

Food that influence organs/meridians: Sweets and Sugar, mucus forming foods (cheese, milk, refined flour products), low fiber amount, acidic foods.

Areas associated with Lungs/Large Intestine: Edema, swelling, hardness, discoloration, temperature changes and abnormalities along lungs and large intestine meridians.

- **The lung meridians (11 tsubos)** begin in the middle burner, solar plexus and travels down to the large intestines. It then travels up past the stomach, it divides into two lines at the diaphragm and over the lungs. It then unites again, going straight up the center front of the neck, separates again, traveling down diagonally to lung one at the pecs just below the anterior deltoid. At that point it passes over the shoulder down the arm along the outer biceps, forearm, wrist, base of the thumb (pollicis) culminating at the outside of the thumbnail.

- **The large intestine meridians (20 tsubos)** begin at the outside (pinky side) corner of the index finger, over the wrist between the thumb and index finger, past the elbow, up arm (triceps), shoulder muscle, across shoulder blade, side of neck, over the cheek, lip, ending at the wings of the nose.

Signs of Imbalance: tightness in chest, difficulty breathing, shortness of breath, shallow breathing, lung disorders (asthma), allergies, cough, dryness, rounding of shoulders, dull skin, pale or puffy cheeks, drooping posture, throat and nasal issues, weak lower back, skin problems (acne), forefinger pain and weak thumb (pollicis muscle), pain along arms and shoulders (L.I. extensors, Lungs. Flexors) forearm, upper arm (biceps, triceps), flexor digitorum, pecs, outer shoulder muscle (deltoid), trapezius, inside front of neck, diaphragm, intestinal imbalances, quadratus lumborum, gluteus medius.

Time of Day (Chinese Clock): The hours for the lung meridian is 3am-5am, the hours for the large intestine meridian is 5am-7am.

Associated Emotion: grief, sadness, detached, depression, self-rejection, feelings of loneliness, lack of confidence, negativity.

Lung Meridian

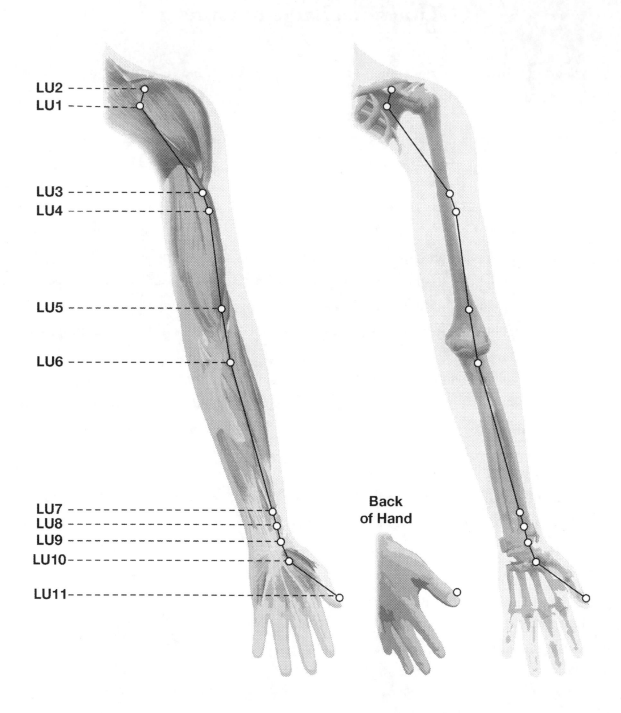

LU2
LU1
LU3
LU4
LU5
LU6
LU7
LU8
LU9
LU10
LU11

Back of Hand

Illustration 30

Large Intestine
(Arm)

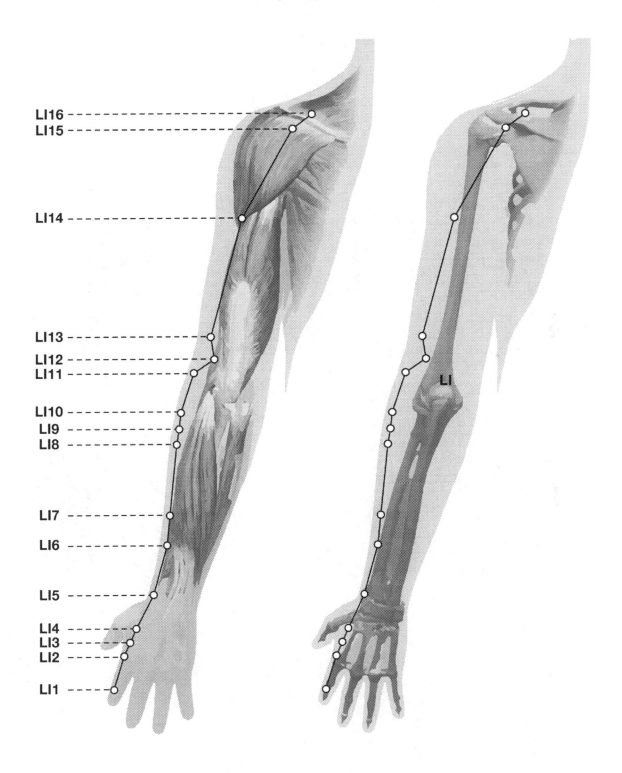

LI16
LI15
LI14
LI13
LI12
LI11
LI10
LI9
LI8
LI7
LI6
LI5
LI4
LI3
LI2
LI1

LI

Illustration 31

Large Intestine
(Head)

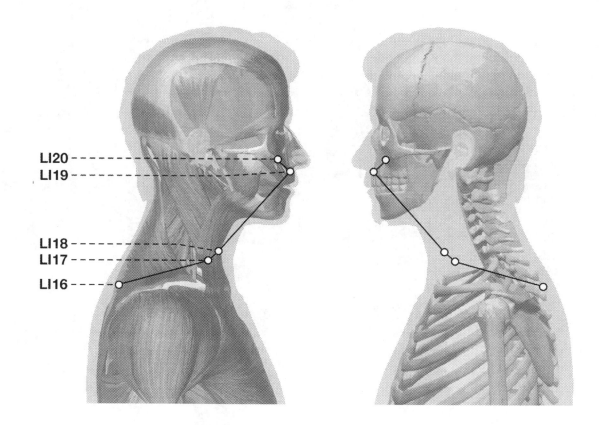

LI20
LI19

LI18
LI17
LI16

Illustration 32

Notes: If you're eating the amount of fiber you should be eating, what you put in your mouth should take 24-48 hours to run out the other side. Fiber is currently a huge issue in the American diet. The average American consumes about half the fiber their body requires. That's an awful lot of people with constipation and eventually intestinal complaints. Since we don't get enough fiber, things go through our body more sluggishly. In fact, if you're very low on fiber, it can take up to two weeks to get out the other end. A low-fiber intake person can theoretically be carrying around a week's worth of food in their gut. If you eat three meals a day, that's 21 meals. We're not getting the fiber to push everything through, so everything just sits and creates inflammation. There's a lot of those animal products that create arachidonic acid, which is a highly inflammatory thing, so if your lower back is always hurting and your hips are inflamed, you need more fiber.

The more fiber you have, the better things move through your body and especially the better your body detoxes and burns calories. You can calculate the amount of fiber you need based on how much you eat. According to the Centers for Disease Control and Prevention, for every thousand calories of intake, you'll need at least 14 grams of fiber. Your height, weight and activity level will also determine how many calories you need. The average women consume about 1,833 calories per day (need about 25 grams of fiber). The average man consumes about 2400 calories (need about 35 grams of fiber). A 120-pound person would require about 25 grams of fiber per day, a larger person, 30 to 35 grams. A large bowl of oatmeal is 8 grams of fiber. So, if you're a guy about my size (170 pounds), you would need to eat four bowls of oatmeal per day. No one is going to do that, yet that's what is required. An apple is 2 grams of fiber, so I would need to eat 15 apples a day to get my fiber. A slice of whole wheat bread is around 2 grams of fiber, so I would need to eat the whole loaf. The problem with bread, even organic whole wheat bread is as soon as you process a whole grain into a flour product, the glycemic index dramatically increases, and the bread turns to sugar very quickly. That's like eating a candy bar. The idea here is that there are not a lot of great sources of fiber. Most people think that fruits and vegetable are fiber (I eat a salad every day, Larry!). But salad is mostly water. There are some veggies that do have significant fiber, like kale or broccoli, but you would have to eat the whole head to get 15 grams! That doesn't get you to your minimum daily requirement of 30 grams of fiber. The truth of this is that if you're eating a grain or a bean at every meal, you're getting the fiber you need.

If you're not, odds are, you're not getting enough fiber, sorry.

Think of it like this: you go to a steak house and they ask how you would like your steak cooked? Rare, medium rare, black and blue, well done?

A lot of people like it on the rare side, so very often that tuna steak or chopped beef, if it's on the rare side, that means it not that well-cooked.

If you count how many times a person chews while they're eating, the average person chews maybe 5, 6, 10 times a mouth-full before they swallow?

Maybe you should be chewing it 35-70 times, and liquefying that particular food, but most don't. So now you're gulping; you're eating all this rare flesh and you're not chewing it well. It goes down into the stomach, but the stomach can only hold it for around 20 minutes because while that meat is supposed to sit in your stomach acid for hours, you have decided to have a glass of ginger ale, which contains sugar. Or a rum and coke, or a white-flour dinner roll that had sugar in the batter. Or an appetizer that was a simple carbohydrate. The rule is, when you put simple carbs in the body, it can only sit in the stomach for a certain amount of time, and then it has to be passed down to the small intestine.

So, in 20 or 30 minutes, all this raw meat gets passed down to the small intestine, and the small intestine calls up the stomach and says,

"What are you doing? I can't digest this, it's all raw, the guy hasn't even chewed! I don't have the digestive enzymes! What happened to the hydrochloric acid??"

The stomach calls back and says, *"I'm sorry. The guy took in all this sugar, all these simple carbs, I gotta pass it through, the law says I gotta pass it through, otherwise I'm gonna have a big problem. So now you gotta figure out what to do with it."*

So now all this raw, undigested food gets passed down to the large intestine eventually, and it's just passing slowly, meandering through, and because you're not eating a lot of fiber, it's just sitting around, and you're getting all this inflammatory response, and you get chronic low back pain. Which, by the way, the whole world has chronic low back pain because nobody eats fiber or chews, and everybody eats too much animal food at this point. Big problem.

So, what would that rare meat look like if it were 104° degrees outside, and we took that piece of rare, partially cooked meat and put it into a plastic bag and closed up the bag and put it out into the 104-degree sun for four or five days?

Whatever is sitting inside that bag is probably what it's looking like sitting inside your intestine after a week. Now if that be the case, that's going to be nasty, and I want to say that is the reason why most people have a deodorant for every orifice of their body at this point. There is a reason why smells are coming out of the parts of our body that it shouldn't. When that person takes off their shoes and socks after a lifetime of eating cows, chickens, lambs, sheep, and pigs—all that dead, putrefying flesh is going to decay, and all that decay is going to smell like death. And that person is a walking animal death camp. And they're wondering why everything smells! These people have body odors, and you know as well as I do, as a massage therapist, when people take their clothes off, it's like thank God I don't have a good sense of smell, because if I have to smell all this...you get the point.

We need fiber to move everything through, and when you get it, you'll have a speeded-up metabolism, you'll burn calories more quickly, you'll do much better.

That's what we want to create.

Now when it comes to your lungs, we need to talk about the mucous forming, sticky foods.

When you eat dairy, cheese in general or drink milk, the phlegmy, sticky stuff that gets caught in the back of your throat is what they make Elmer's Glue out of.

Elmer's glue is made by the Borden's dairy company with a little picture of Elsie the cow in the upper left corner.

Dairy is the number one food allergy food on the planet Earth. The reason is obvious.

You are not a cow.

A baby calf is 60 pounds at birth and grows to be 1600 pounds in just two years!

That's an awful lot of growth in just two years.

Took you many more years than that.

That mommy cow's milk for baby must be super rich and filled with some very serious growth hormones.

Stuff I don't want to put in my family's body at all.

In addition, it takes ten pounds of milk to make one pound of cheese.

Hardened, concentrated, saturated glue.

Now back to the lungs…

Flour products have traditionally been used to make paste.

When I was a kid in kindergarten, when you ran out of Elmer's Glue, you made paste out of flour and water.

Both dairy products and flour products will glue up your lungs, your intestines, and contribute to all sorts of different problems from allergies and asthma, digestive problems, cancers, heart disease, diabetes.

Water Element

Kidneys and Bladder

Bladder, kidneys, adrenals, reproductive.

Food that influence organs/meridians: animal foods, cheap table salt, over consumption of water or not enough, poor quality drinking water (reverse osmosis, distillation), chlorination/ fluoridation, excess stimulants (sugar, tea, coffee, alcohol, hot spice, excess tropical), excess baked goods, cold food and drinks (ice), avoid acidic-producing foods.

Areas associated with Kidneys/Bladder: Edema, swelling, hardness, discoloration, temperature changes and abnormalities along kidney and bladder meridians.

- **The kidney meridians (27 tsubos)** begin at the bottom of the foot, specifically the indentation made when you curl the toes forward, traveling around the ankle, up the in side of the leg, inside of knee on the fatty bursar, up inside of thigh, up to the tip of the coccyx, through the lower abdomen traveling one and a half centimeters to either side of the anterior center line. Alongside the belly button, the meridian goes to the kidneys, then splits one branch to the bladder and the other branch straight up liver, diaphragm and to the lungs. The energy line makes one more split at the lungs, one branch going to the tongue root, the other in the heart and connecting with the heart governor meridian at conception vessel 17, right between the nipples.
- **The bladder meridians (67 tsubos)** are the longest meridians in the human body. They start at the inner portion of the eyelid called eyebright and travel up the front of the head to the back of the head. The meridians then form two branches traveling down the neck, the back, to the sacrum along the spine, along the middle of the butt, and then to the back of the thigh, meeting behind the knee and traveling along the calf, the Achilles tendon to the outside of the foot. The meridian ends at the outside of the pinky toe.

Signs of Imbalance: cramps in back of legs, weak willpower, insecure, aloof, isolated, tight, hard, cold over kidneys or bladder, shoes wear on angle outside, anterior tilt to the waist, lordosis, frown lines over kidneys on back, bow-legged, leg cramps, bouncing legs, swollen feet, edema, low back pain over kidneys, eye disease, bags under eyes, dark color under or around eyes, wet hands, leaning forward while sitting, standing or walking indicates tight yang kidneys,

Kidney Meridian
(Back of Legs)

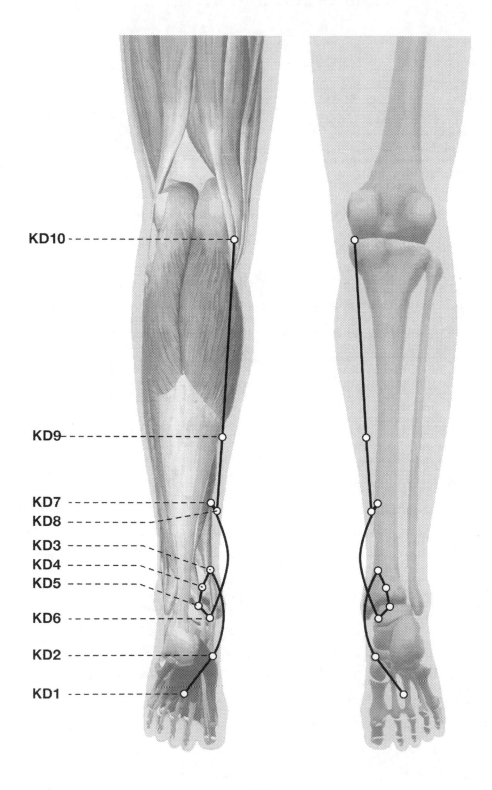

KD10

KD9

KD7
KD8
KD3
KD4
KD5
KD6
KD2
KD1

Illustration 33

Kidney Meridian
(Torso)

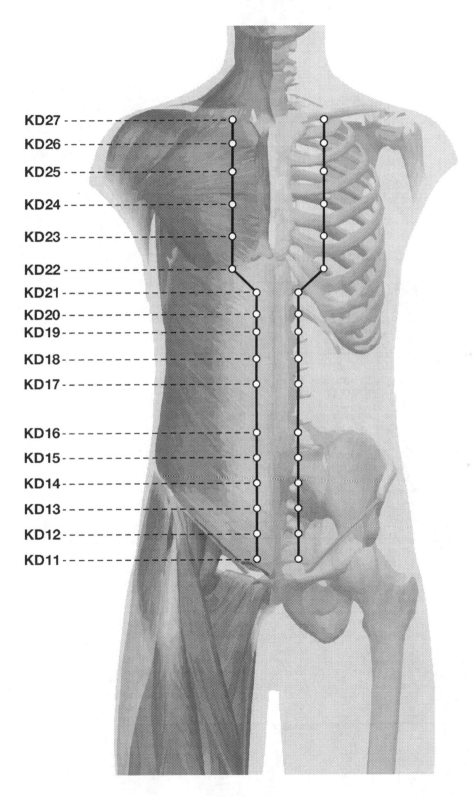

KD27
KD26
KD25
KD24
KD23
KD22
KD21
KD20
KD19
KD18
KD17

KD16
KD15
KD14
KD13
KD12
KD11

Illustration 34

Bladder Meridian
(Back and Head)

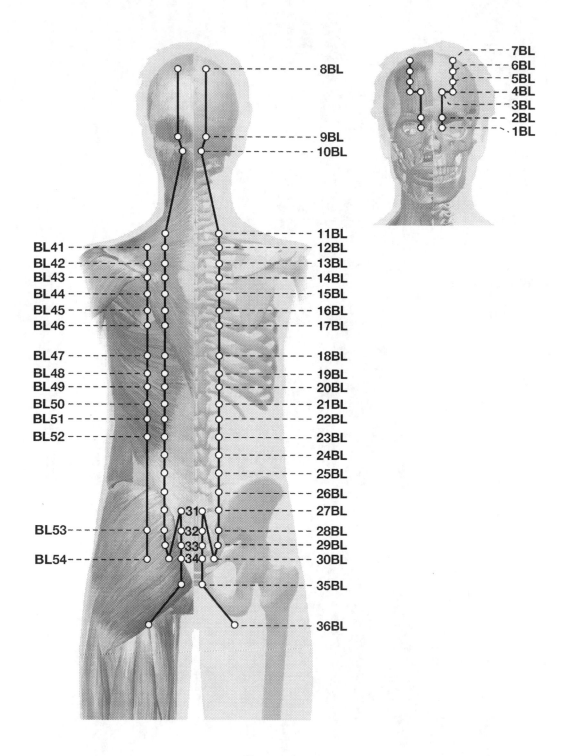

Illustration 35

Bladder Meridian
(Back of Legs and Foot)
All point should be referenced with BL prefix

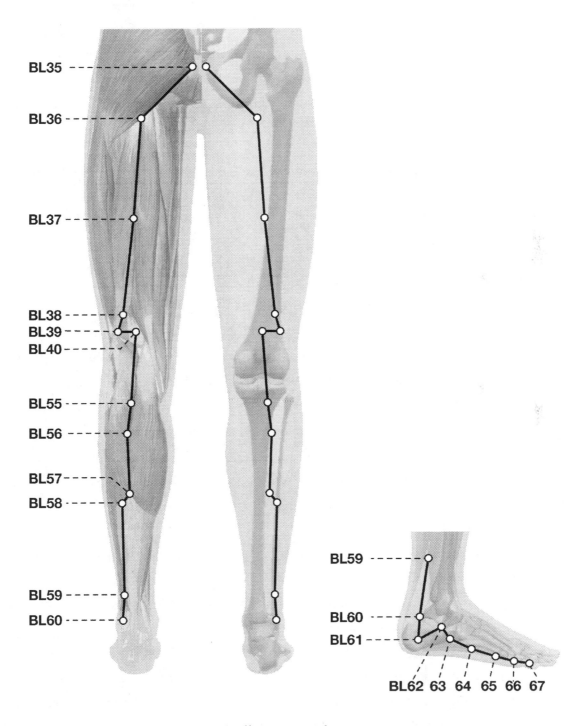

Illustration 36

slouching, leaning yin expanded kidneys, fatigue, low energy, overall weakness, lack of vitality, signs of acid: dry, itchy skin, infection ie. candida, yeast, athlete's foot, flu, ear infection, frequent urination, urinary incontinence, night sweats, poor short-term memory, low back pain, hearing loss, ringing in the ears, osteoporosis, sexual dysfunction, dark and rough complexion, poor memory, inability to think clearly, and backache are all regarded as indicators of impaired kidney function and deficient kidney energy, groove created in bottom of foot when toes are in flexion (kidney 1), inside of ankle (kidney points), lateral foot to pinky toe (bladder line), the pinky toe itself (bladder), Achilles tendon, back of calves, back of thighs (hamstrings), area directly over kidneys and/or bladder, glutes, erector spinae group, eyes, psoas, iliacus, peroneals.

Condition influences: emotional stress, fear, terror, lack of sleep, acidic blood stream, adrenaline events

Time of Day (Chinese Clock): The hours for bladder are 3 to 5 p.m.; kidney is 5 to 7 p.m.

Associated Emotion: fear, mis-trust, paranoia, depression, anxiety, lack of self-respect, timidity, hopelessness

Notes: When we eat too much animal protein, the kidneys are overworked. Our kidneys in an attempt to detox the excess, involuntarily bounce the legs up and down.

On my honeymoon, we went to an all-inclusive in Aruba where one of the restaurants was a grill type of place. Since the grilled food and beverage was included in the costs, everyone ate and drank heavily. Then an amazing thing was noticed. Everyone in the place, at one time was bouncing their legs—the whole place!!

One big detox. I took out my phone and took a video of the bouncing legs. I still have it.

There are two main types of kidney problems.

Tight, contracted kidneys: This condition restricts free flow of blood; caused used by excess sodium, animal foods, salty foods (cheese, canned tuna), baked food and can be exacerbated by a stressful busy lifestyle.

Swollen, loose kidneys: Caused by excess liquid, fruits, juice, alcohol, stimulants (caffeine etc.), inactive lifestyle.

Kidney disease is in the top ten causes of death. This is caused by excess protein. When you consume protein loads all the time, it wears out the kidneys.

When a person is young, they tell you to drink a lot of water. Just flush your body with water. But when you get old and have kidney problems or congestive heart failure, they limit your water to avoid overworking your kidneys and heart. So, a lot in one case, and a little in the other. In Oriental medicine, they say to drink when you're thirsty because drinking lots of water will wear out your kidneys and body. That's the opposite of how we think in America, but perhaps there's a reason for the American version. If you eat the model American diet, bacon and eggs for breakfast, ham and cheese for lunch, meatloaf and mashed potatoes for dinner with a bowl of ice cream for dessert, you better drink a lot of water!

Did you ever notice how small the teacups are in Japanese and Chinese culture?

Here, we get a big mug of coffee or tea.

It's not because the Asian culture is inhospitable.

It's because they're paying attention.

All living things suffer terribly from pain and want desperately to live.

The more evolved mammals, such as monkeys, pigs, cows, dogs, to name a few, due to their awareness and sentience, perhaps even more so.

At the moment of slaughter and death, they emit tremendous fear chemicals into their bloodstreams and their flesh, just like you do.

Unfortunately, that's what you feed your children or yourself in a hamburger.

So, if what you reap, is what you sow and every action has an equal and opposite reaction, then those that cause pain will receive pain in return.

Unfortunately, it catches up to you in a myriad of ways, not just when you are old, although that's probably the worst.

There's a reason why more than half of America is on anti-depressives.

Remember what Buddha said,

"Cause no suffering."

Think about it and make some changes.

And God said, Behold, I have given you every herb bearing seed, which is upon the face of all the earth, and every tree, in the which is the fruit of a tree yielding seed; to you it shall be for meat.

Genesis 1:29 (KJV)

Wood Element

Liver and Gall Bladder

Food that influence organs/meridians: animal fats (meat, cheese), alcohol, vinegar, eggs, over-eating, over the counter medications, chemical exposure, statin drugs, obesity.

Areas associated with Liver/Gall Bladder: Edema, swelling, hardness, discoloration, temperature changes and abnormalities along liver and bladder meridians.

- **The liver meridian (14 tsubos)** starts on the inside of the big toenail, goes between the big toe and second, travels in front of the inside ankle and up the inside of the leg. It continues upwards, passes the knee, continues along the adductors into the groin area, then into the lower abdomen moving on to both the liver and gall bladder, then ribs, the throat, to the eye, and ends on top of the crown of the head.
- **The gall bladder meridian (44 tsubos)** begins outside the corner of the eye, turns down then around the ear, up to the forehead just within the hair line, descends behind the ear to the corner of the skull, back to the forehead above the center of the eye, moves down the head to the bottom of the skull, continuing down the neck to the shoulder, travels the side of the body along the ribs, to the waist, pelvis, continuing down the peroneals, to the ankle, ending on the outside of the 4th toe.

Signs of Imbalance: insomnia- waking up suddenly, very early in the morning and not being able to fall asleep again, tendons, eye complaints, glaucoma, tight neck, dizziness, headaches, tendonitis, PMS, mood swings, tearing eyes and tears, high shoulder, rib on right side high or displaced, interscapular knot on right side, tight, hard, cold on upper right quadrant of back, outside of ankle, sides of hips (IT Band), sides of calves (peroneus longus, brevis and tertius), stiffness in muscles and joints; stiff shoulders; hips or neck, eye problems, emotional imbalance. Also, these muscles can be affected; anterior deltoids, pec major, serratus anterior, lats, rhomboids, peroneus muscles, IT Band, adductors, inside and outside of knee, inside calf, inside thigh, swelling and pain on the fourth toe where the gall bladder meridian begins.

Time of Day (Chinese Clock): the hours for the gall bladder is 11pm to 1am, the hours for the liver is 1am-3am.

Liver Meridian

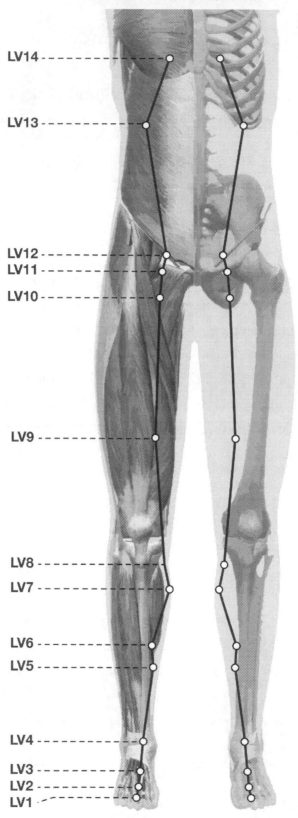

LV14

LV13

LV12
LV11

LV10

LV9

LV8
LV7

LV6
LV5

LV4

LV3
LV2
LV1

Illustration 37

Gall Bladder Meridian

All point should be referenced with GB prefix

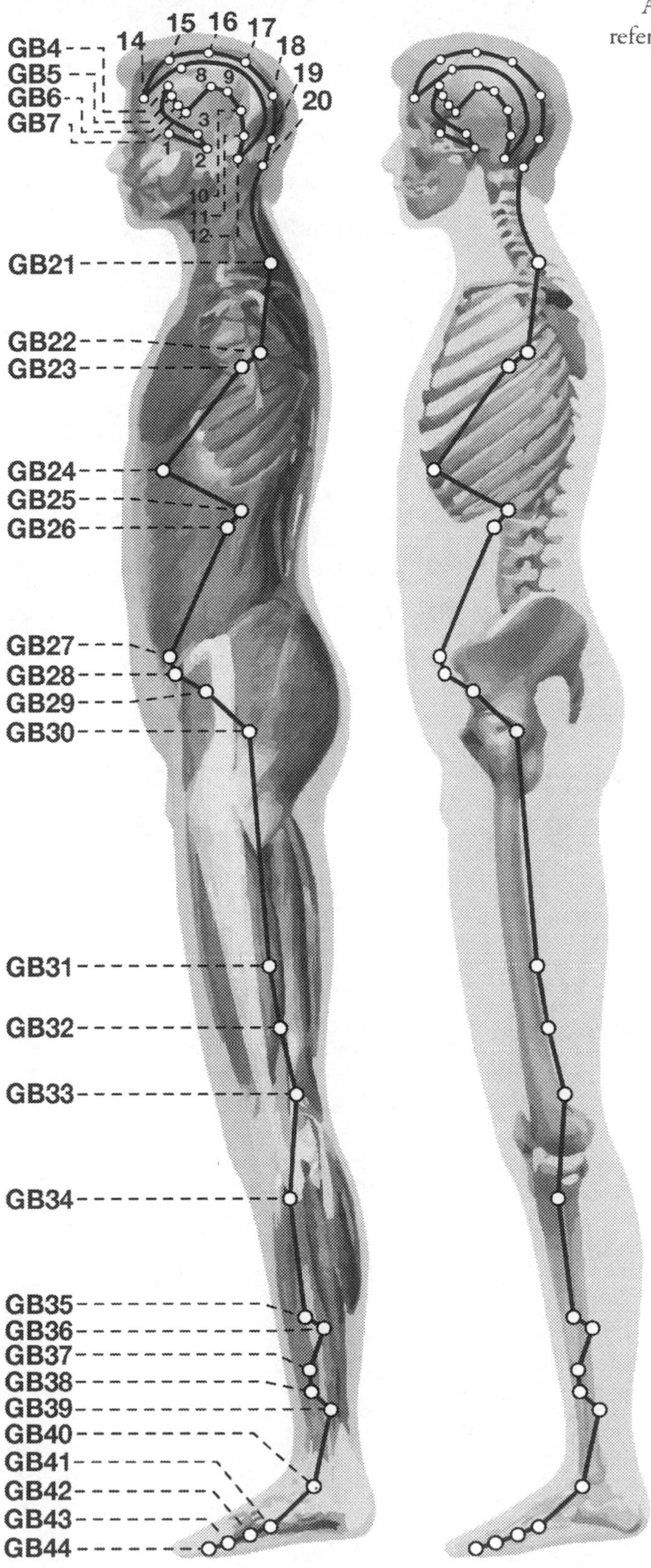

GB4
GB5
GB6
GB7
14 15 16 17 18 19 20
8 9
3
1 2
10
11
12

GB21

GB22
GB23

GB24
GB25
GB26

GB27
GB28
GB29
GB30

GB31

GB32

GB33

GB34

GB35
GB36
GB37
GB38
GB39
GB40
GB41
GB42
GB43
GB44

Illustration 38

Emotion associated: anger, frustration, anxiety, resentment, frustration, irritability, bitterness, "flying off the handle," impatience, rage, aggression, violent thoughts and acts

Notes: These meridians affect most Americans. You can tell when a person has a liver or gall bladder issues: You're driving down Rt. 46, you're getting closer and closer to the intersection, an on-coming car is waiting to make a turn at the intersection, they wait until you're almost there, then mosey out into the lane. They're going 20 mph, and you're coming at around 45 mph. You start to scream "Why couldn't you just wait? Why were you so impatient? Can't people just wait another second? Why cut me off? What were you thinking?" But they weren't thinking, and they just had a big double cheese pizza, with some sort of soda beverage, and their liver is completely overworked, and they're impatient, and angry and think they have a right to whatever, and that's the problem.

It's easy to have a chemical exposure; just look under your kitchen counter at all the disinfectants and cleaners. These are some of the basic things that affect liver and gall bladder. If there is a large excess of these foods that you consume, then it might affect the organ associated with that meridian, and those muscles would be affected.

How To Use This Information

This is just the beginning.

There are more questions, than answers.

There are so many possibilities, so many avenues when it comes to our human body.

Functional soft tissue work addresses the symptoms and looks for the causes.

Is it nutrition, genetics, overuse, psychology?

Actually, it's all of it.

My intention for writing this book is to shake things up and encourage us to

consider a larger picture, one that tries to identify the causes.

A Massage Grandmaster's Soft Tissue Rules

The Rules are:

- our first job as massage therapists is to break up the hardness!
- find the hard, cold areas and you'll find the problems.
- anything that increases circulation, decreases pain. That's why heat, ice and even magnets can work.
- when you eat more than your body can burn the excess has to be stored or discharged. It must go somewhere.
- you always palpate and treat an area by starting lightly at the point of resistance, then you slowly desensitize the area as if you were peeling an onion one layer at a time.
- cause no pain.
- every time you ask a prospective client where it hurts, consider you are addressing pulled, torn or damaged muscle tissue like sprains and strains.
- the strongest energy comes off the fingertips.
- pain in an acu-point or a region can indicate imbalance or blockage energetically in an organ or its energetic system.
- always wear good support on your feet when giving massage (otherwise you can shorten your career and wear out your body).
- whether you are treating trigger points or acu-points, treat all points a minimum of 8 seconds.
- whenever you want to activate a treatment point, hit it, repeatedly over an over again. Successful activation will take considerable patience.
- your body positioning is a crucial component for a long career. No slumped shoulders or crossed legs. Clean, straight lines.
- we address all complaints with an arsenal of techniques but there are about 15 soft tissue complaints that we absolutely excel at. Soft tissue complaints respond best to soft tissue solutions. It cannot be addressed in short increments. The therapist must work an entire region culminating in the specific spot. It will take time. I have my greatest success with a 90-minute session.
- shiatsu and acupressure work better if you break up the muscular armoring first.
- to make and keep a complete electrical connection, always keep both hands on the body
- if in doubt, leave it out!

Bibliography

1. https://www.ncbi.nlm.nih.gov/pmc/articles/PMC3838801
   Proof that acupuncture meridians exist. NIH in 2013

2. The Journal of Orthopaidic and Sports Physical Therapy Copyright 1982 by The Orthopaedic and Sports Physical Therapy Sections of the American Physical Therapy Association Cyriax's Friction Massage: A Review Gail J. Chamberlain, MA, PT*

3. Järvinen MJ, Lehto MU The effects of early mobilization and immobilization on the healing process following muscle injuries.

4. Sports Med (Auckland, N.Z.), 15 (2) (1993), pp. 78-89
   Blasier RB, Morawa LG. Complete rupture of the hamstring origin from a water-skiing injury. Am J Sports Med. 18(4):435-7

5. https://www.ncbi.nlm.nih.gov/pmc/articles/PMC4003788/
   Role of Serum Fibrinogen Levels in Patients with Rotator Cuff Tears

6. https://www.ncbi.nlm.nih.gov/pmc/articles/PMC4767755
   Current concept of spleen-stomach theory and spleen deficiency syndrome in TCM

7. https://www.jospt.org/doi/pdf/10.2519/jospt.1982.4.1.16
   https://www.ncbi.nlm.nih.gov/pmc/articles/PMC3838801

8. Evid Based Complement Alternat Med. 2013; 2013: 739293.
   Wave-Induced Flow in Meridians Demonstrated Using Photoluminescent Bioceramic Material on Acupuncture Points
   C. Will Chen, 1 Chen-Jei Tai, 2, 3 Cheuk-Sing Choy, 4 Chau-Yun Hsu, 5 Shoei-Loong Lin, 6, 7 Wing P. Chan, 8, 9 Han-Sun Chiang, 10 Chang-An Chen, 11 and Ting-Kai Leung 8, 9, 12, 13,*

9. http://www.earthsave.org/environment.htm

10. Lester Brown, et al., Vital Signs 1994 (Washington, DC: Worldwatch Institute, 1994)

11. Robert Repetto "Renewable Resources and Population Growth," Population and Environment 10:4 (Summer 1989) pg. 228-29 cited in Rifkin, Beyond Beef (New York: Dutton Press, 1992).

12. Tom Aldridge and Herb Schlubach, "Water Requirements for Food Production," Soil and Water, no. 38 (Fall 1978), University of California Cooperative Extension, 13017; Paul and Anne Ehrlich, Population, Resources, Environment (San Francisco: Freemna, 1972), pg. 75-76

13. Peter Egoscue, The Egoscue Method of Health Through Motion, Harper, 1992

14. Robert J. Stone, Atlas of the Skeletal Muscles, Wm.C.Brown Publishers, 1990

15. Bonnie Prudden, Pain Erasure, The Bonnie Prudden Way, M. Evans & Company, 1980

16. Janet G. Travell, M.D. and David G. Simons, M.D., Myofascial Pain and Dysfunction, The Trigger Point Manual, Williams& Wilkins, 1992

17. Michio Kushi and Alex Jack, The Macrobiotic Path To Total Health, Ballantine Books, 2003

18. Michio Kushi, How To see Your Health: Book of Oriental Diagnosis, Japan Publications, 1980

19. Masahiro Oki, Zen Yoga Therapy, Japan Publications, 1979

20. Ye-Seul Lee, 1 Yeonhee Ryu, 2 Won-Mo Jung, 1 Jungjoo Kim, 1 Taehyung Lee, 1 and Younbyoung Chae, Understanding Mind-Body Interaction from the Perspective of East Asian Medicine, Evid Based Complement Alternat Med. 2017; 2017: 7618419.

21. Sports Medicine Australia, https://sma.org.au/resources-advice/injury-fact-sheets

22. https://en.wikipedia.org/wiki/Bonnie_Prudden

23. http://www.myotherapy.org/roots.php

24. https://erikdalton.com/blog/protective-muscle-spasm

25. https://www.ncbi.nlm.nih.gov/pmc/articles/PMC4456393/ Risk Factors and Disability Associated with Low Back Pain in Older Adults in Low- and Middle-Income Countries. Results from the WHO Study on Global AGEing and Adult Health (SAGE

26. https://news.curtin.edu.au/media-releases/conditions-like-back-pain-arthritis-must-global-health-response
    May edition of Bulletin of the World Health Organization (WHO),
    https://www.ncbi.nlm.nih.gov/pmc/articles/PMC2572532/
    Bull World Health Organ. 2003; 81(9): 671–676.
    Published online 2003 Nov 14.
    PMCID: PMC2572532
    PMID: 14710509
    Low back pain.
    George E. Ehrlich

27. http://myheart.net/earlobe-crease-and-heart-disease-fact-or-myth

About The Author
Larry Heisler, M.A., LMT

One of New Jersey's massage therapy pioneers (since 1975), Larry Heisler, M.A., LMT is the founder and director of the longest running massage school in the Garden State, the North Jersey Massage Training Center. Larry has taught massage therapy to thousands of students and has dramatically affected the massage and bodywork landscape in the tri-state region. Larry became Director of Nutrition for the Parsippany Medical Complex after attending two alternative nutrition programs; the Kushi Institute and the Donsbach School of Nutrition. It was at the K.I. that Larry learned how to combine the macrobiotic nutritional counseling with traditional barefoot shiatsu. In fact, the first 8,000 massages Larry performed were entirely traditional barefoot shiatsu. Larry's skills were so dynamic, that within a few years he had a substantial clientele and dozens of students apprenticing with him.

By the mid-eighties, Larry had a full-fledged massage therapy program with a cutting-edge curriculum combining a fusion of Eastern and Western medical massage applications. His revolutionary approach to bodywork is based on the direct influence the acupuncture meridian system has on the human musculature. Larry's school has been widely acknowledged for its volunteer massage team participation in many hundreds of state-wide fund-raising events for organizations like the Cystic Fibrosis Foundation, Muscular Dystrophy, the Diabetes Foundation, the Red Cross, the Leukemia Society, Make A Wish Foundation, Multiple Sclerosis Foundation and the 9/11 Port Authority Ground Zero Command to name just a few. Larry was one of the very first in New Jersey to present what is now called Integrative Medical Programs in Wellness, Nutrition, Massage and Meditation for the hospital medical staffs at six different Grand Medical Rounds Symposiums including the New Jersey School of Medicine and Dentistry. Each one of those hospitals began offering Integrative Medicine divisions after Larry's presentations. In addition, Larry's school created and conducted the very first hospital-based massage therapy program offered in NJ. He also created a massage organization entitled, the United Bodywork and Massage Practitioners of NJ. At that time, his group was as large as the NJ Chapter of AMTA and was directly created to even the playing field and prevent the American Massage Therapy Association from enacting an exclusive Swedish massage license they were heavily promoting. To stop that monopoly from occurring Larry had an all-inclusive massage certification bill created specifically by a professional bill writer in the N.Y. Legislature. That became the model for a fair and just certification bill in the Garden State. His personal activism culminated on television with then Governor Christie Todd Whitman, where the Governor made it clear that a bodywork monopoly would not be tolerated. Larry's United Bodywork organization then became one of the founding member groups of the Associated Bodywork and Massage Professionals. In addition, Larry has presented programs on over thirty college campuses, for a dozen health departments, for a hundred different religious organizations, at many hundreds of New Jersey/New York corporations, has written the holistic wellness curriculum for three Universities and has done dozens of popular radio health shows like the Gary Null Show.

Currently, Larry's school offers classes to improve the competitive skills of already licensed practitioners by offering advanced education on a continuing education basis. In fact, Larry's school is one of the major continuing education providers in the tri-state region. And while dozens of highly qualified educators share their talents at his school, Larry personally offers over a dozen classes himself. There are thousands upon thousands of glowing evaluations on file at the school written by students after taking Larry's classes. Whenever you see therapists using a rocking elbow technique to the posterior body, chances are they studied with Larry.

In massage and bodywork, Larry is considered a Grand-Master, having personally treated an estimated 60,000 patients including thousands of world class athletes. His email newsletter goes out to 9,000 massage therapists and he has an exclusive arrangement for his school to offer Certification in Manual Lymph Drainage from the prestigious Manual Lymph Drainage Institute. Larry believes MLD will change the entire massage profession! Aside from his extensive education in massage therapy, Larry holds additional degree's and certifications in counseling, nutrition, education and ministry.

Larry wants to personally thank his wife, children, and office staff for their continued support and unconditional love and lastly his teachers, meditation master Hilda Charlton, Sensei's Michio Kushi, Masahiro Oki, Shizuko Yamamoto, Dr. Wally Burnstein, and Ingeborg Schlobohm, LMT.

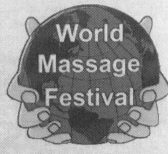

World Massage Festival

World Massage Festival

hereby inducts

Larry Heisler

into the 2019

Massage Therapy Hall of Fame

in recognition

of his contributions to the art and science of

Massage Therapy

May 6-9, 2019   *Mike Hinkle, Founder*

Printed in the United States
By Bookmasters